Modern Management of Obstructive Sleep Apnea

Salam O. Salman
Editor

Modern Management of Obstructive Sleep Apnea

Springer

Editor
Salam O. Salman
Oral and Maxillofacial Surgery
University of Florida – Jacksonville
Jacksonville, FL
USA

ISBN 978-3-030-11442-8 ISBN 978-3-030-11443-5 (eBook)
https://doi.org/10.1007/978-3-030-11443-5

Library of Congress Control Number: 2019935901

This Springer imprint is published by the registered company Springer Nature Switzerland AG
The registered company address is: Gewerbestrasse 11, 6330 Cham, Switzerland

Contents

1 Medical Evaluation of Patients with Obstructive Sleep Apnea

Scott Steinberg and Mariam Louis

1.1 Introduction

Obstructive sleep apnea (OSA), defined as repetitive collapse of the upper airway during sleep leading to intermittent hypoxia and frequent arousals from sleep, is the most common sleep-related breathing disorder that represents a global health concern. Many countries have the same, if not higher, prevalence of OSA than in the USA [1, 2]. With the obesity pandemic on the rise, the number of OSA cases can be expected to increase with it. The identification and appropriate diagnosis of OSA are important because of the medical consequences associated with untreated disease. Hypertension, cardiovascular morbidity, neurocognitive decline, diabetes, and a metabolic syndrome are all potential sequela of untreated OSA. Perioperative and overall mortality is increased as well. Here we will discuss the risk factors, clinical presentation of OSA, and the methods used to diagnose it. Polysomnography is the gold standard test for identifying sleep-disordered breathing (SDB) as well as assessing its severity and the efficacy of therapy with positive airway pressure (PAP) devices.

1.2 Epidemiology and Risk Factors

The prevalence of OSA varies dependent on the definitions used by various epidemiologic investigators. The Wisconsin Sleep Cohort Study, published in 1993, defined SDB as an AHI ≥ 5. Sleep apnea syndrome was present when the AHI was ≥ 5, and symptoms of hypersomnolence were present. The prevalence of SDB was 9% in middle-aged women and 24% in middle-aged men. The prevalence of sleep

S. Steinberg · M. Louis (✉)
Division of Pulmonary, Critical Care and Sleep Medicine, Department of Medicine, College of Medicine, University of Florida—Jacksonville, Jacksonville, FL, USA
e-mail: scott.steinberg@jax.ufl.edu; mariam.louis@jax.ufl.edu

S. O. Salman (ed.), *Modern Management of Obstructive Sleep Apnea*,
https://doi.org/10.1007/978-3-030-11443-5_1

apnea syndrome on the other hand was 4% in middle-aged men and 2% in middle-aged women [3]. More current studies show higher estimates ranging from 15 to 30% in men and 5 to 15% in women [4–6]. This increase in prevalence parallels the rising rates of obesity, although improved technology and better detection likely play a role as well.

The prevalence of OSA increases from young adulthood through the sixth and seventh decade of life, at which point it plateaus. In addition, racial and ethnic differences in OSA prevalence have been identified. It is more prevalent in young African Americans when compared to Caucasians of the same age, independent of body weight [7]. These differences may in part be due to craniofacial and upper airway abnormalities that lead to an abnormal or constricted maxilla or small mandibular size, a wide craniofacial base, and tonsillar and adenoid hypertrophy. It should be noted that while the latter plays an important role in pediatric OSA, its contribution to OSA in adults is substantially less. Other recognized risk factors for OSA include nasal congestion, current smoking, and postmenopausal status. Certain medical conditions can also increase the risk of OSA. These include pregnancy, congestive heart failure, end-stage renal disease, stroke, acromegaly, hypothyroidism, polycystic ovary syndrome, and Down syndrome.

1.3 Clinical Presentation

The diagnosis of OSA begins with identifying the signs and symptoms of OSA and developing a clinical suspicion. The clinical features of OSA can be divided into nighttime and daytime symptoms. Nighttime symptoms include snoring, gasping, or choking during sleep, nocturia, frequent arousals from sleep/insomnia, dry mouth, and morning headaches. Daytime symptoms include daytime sleepiness, fatigue, nonrestorative sleep, poor concentration, irritability, decreased libido, and obesity. It should be noted that some patients with severe OSA may have minimal daytime symptoms, so a high index of suspicion is needed.

The physical examination for OSA will usually reveal an elevated BMI as well as a crowded upper airway. Vital signs should include blood pressure and BMI. Determining the Mallampati score can help identify narrow upper airways. In addition, tonsillar size and facial anomalies, such as a small midface, retrognathia, high-arched palate, and so forth, should be noted, as they are a risk factors for OSA. Neck circumference should be measured with values ≥17 in. in men and ≥16 in. in women being a risk factor [8].

Clinical probability tools have been developed to aid clinicians when there is a clinical suspicion for OSA. However, it has been only validated in highly symptomatic patients with a high probability of having OSA and should not be used as a screening tool in asymptomatic patients. The most common sleep questionnaire used in the perioperative setting is the STOP-BANG questionnaire, which has been shown to have the highest sensitivity [9]. Other questionnaires include the sleep apnea clinical score (SACS), the Berlin questionnaire, the NoSAS score, and the multivariable apnea prediction instrument (MVAP). Objective testing is indicated in patients with unexplained excessive daytime sleepiness. In the absence of excessive daytime sleepiness, the presence of snoring plus two other clinical features of OSA should be evaluated with objective testing.

1.4 Complications and Consequences

Many adverse health outcomes have been associated with untreated OSA. Due to increased arousal events and sleep fragmentation, sleep with OSA is generally less restorative, resulting in excessive daytime sleepiness and fatigue. Drowsy driving is common, and motor vehicle collisions occur more frequently among patients with OSA [10]. There may be cognitive and psychiatric findings as well. Observational studies have shown a twofold increased incidence of depression compared to matched controls without OSA [11, 12].

OSA is also a significant risk factor for cardiovascular disease and is associated with increased cardiovascular morbidity and mortality [10–14]. Hypertension is very common and is thought to be associated with increased sympathetic activity during sleep which causes an increase in the release of catecholamines [4]. Treating OSA with PAP has been shown to reduce systolic blood pressures (SBP) but only modestly. Despite the small improvements that are seen in studies, the reductions are still regarded as clinically significant based on studies showing that reductions in SBP of only 1–2 mmHg are associated with reduced cardiovascular events [15]. There is also a significant association between OSA and atrial fibrillation independent of other risk factors. In one study of 400 patients, the incidence of atrial fibrillation on a 24-h Holter monitor was threefold higher than would be expected in the general public [16]. Sleep-disordered breathing is common in patients with heart failure, and OSA may be underdiagnosed in this population since many of the symptoms of OSA could be attributed to heart failure. They may also experience Cheyne-Stokes breathing, which is a type of central apnea common in patients with heart failure.

OSA and diabetes mellitus (DM) are frequently linked as well. Studies have shown that as much as 87% of obese patients with type 2 DM had clinically important OSA [17]. Likewise, longitudinal studies suggest that OSA is a risk factor for DM and diabetic complications [13]. This may be because both conditions have obesity as a primary risk factor; however independent associations have been shown in several large cross-sectional studies [14].

Obstructive sleep apnea also seems to confer a significantly increased risk of developing perioperative complications [18, 19]. The risk varies dependent on the type of surgery; timing of OSA diagnosis, whether it is being treated; and the use of opiates in the postoperative period. Respiratory complications are most common and range from desaturations to ARDS and respiratory failure. Increased rates of cardiovascular complications such as arrhythmias, blood pressure fluctuations, myocardial infarction, and cardiac arrest are also seen [18–20]. The association between OSA and perioperative mortality is unclear. All-cause mortality is increased in patients with severe OSA that is untreated [21, 22].

1.5 Diagnosis

In-laboratory polysomnography is the test of choice for the diagnosis OSA. Polysomnography is a technical exam that monitors several physiologic parameters throughout the night as a patient sleeps. The sleep stages are recorded with an electroencephalogram. Information about eye movements and muscle tone are provided by the electrooculogram and submental electromyography. Respiratory effort is measured via respiratory inductive plethysmography. Nasal prongs measure inspiratory and expiratory airflow, and occasionally end-tidal carbon dioxide monitors are used as an adjunct for identifying hypoventilation. Microphones are utilized to detect snoring, and pulse oximetry is used to monitor the oxygen saturation. Finally, electrocardiography is performed to monitor for the occurrence of arrhythmias during sleep. Other variables such as body position and limb movements are documented as well. The primary outcome measure of polysomnography is the apnea-hypopnea index (AHI). The AHI represents the number of times a patient has cessation of airflow (apnea) or an abnormal reduction in airflow (hypopnea) per hour of sleep. The AHI, used in conjunction with the clinical picture, is diagnostic but also useful for grading the severity of the disease. Full-night or split-night protocols are available, and while full-night testing is only diagnostic, the split-night protocol offers the ability to perform CPAP titration the same night, if the previous portion was diagnostic for OSA. While polysomnography provides a lot of information and the patient is monitored, it is costly and disruptive to the patient. As a result, many insurance companies are authorizing home sleep studies.

Home sleep apnea testing (HSAT) is available and has been shown to be as good as an in-laboratory study for some patients [23]. HSAT is most appropriate for patients with a high pretest probability of having moderate to severe OSA without other significant comorbidities (e.g., moderate-severe pulmonary disorders, neuromuscular diseases, heart disease, neurological disorders, etc.) or sleep disorders (narcolepsy, REM behavioral sleep disorder, etc.). As HSAT cannot verify that the data collected is from a specific individual, patients with mission-critical occupations (an airline pilot, for instance) are not appropriate candidates for HSAT. While HSAT offers convenience and cost benefits, there are important limitations as well. Because fewer physiologic parameters are measured with HSAT, the AHI may be underestimated leading to more false negatives. When clinical suspicion remains high with a negative HSAT, in-laboratory polysomnography should be performed [24]. HSAT is also useful in CPAP titrations and determining efficacy of prescribed therapy.

Nocturnal desaturations documented with overnight pulse oximetry alone are insufficient to make a diagnosis of OSA.

Upon completion of a sleep study, severity of sleep-disordered breathing is best quantified by the patient's AHI. An AHI of <5 is considered normal in the adult population. AHI of 5–15 with associated hypersomnolent symptoms is considered mild, 15–30 moderate, and >30 severe. Other variables, such as positional apnea and lowest oxygen saturation, are important to evaluate as treatment modalities have varying success rates based on those factors, as well as overall severity determined by AHI.

1.6 Summary

Obstructive sleep apnea (OSA) is the most common sleep-related breathing disorder that represents a global health concern. Its prevalence continues to increase in the USA and abroad. The identification and appropriate diagnosis of OSA is crucial due to the multitude of medical sequelae related to untreated OSA. Polysomnography remains the gold standard test for identifying sleep-disordered breathing (SDB) as well as assessing its severity and the efficacy of therapy with positive airway pressure (PAP) devices or surgical interventions.

References

1. Sharma SK, Ahluwalia G. Epidemiology of adult obstructive sleep apnea syndrome in India. Indian J Med Res. 2010;131:171–5.
2. Ip MS, Lam B, Lauder IJ, et al. A community study of sleep-disordered breathing in middle-aged Chinese men in Hong Kong. Chest. 2001;119:62–9.
3. Young T, Palta M, Dempsey J, Skatrud J, Weber S, Badr S. The occurrence of sleep-disordered breathing among middle-aged adults. N Engl J Med. 1993;32:1230–5.
4. Young T, Palta M, Dempsey J, et al. Burden of sleep apnea: rationale, design, and major findings of the Wisconsin sleep cohort study. WMJ. 2009;108:246.
5. Peppard PE, Young T, Barnet JH, et al. Increased prevalence of sleep-disordered breathing in adults. Am J Epidemiol. 2013;177:1006.
6. Dempsey JA, Veasey SC, Morgan BJ, O'Donnel CP. Pathophysiology of sleep apnea. Physiol Rev. 2010;90:47.
7. Redline S, Tishler PV, Hans MG, et al. Racial differences in sleep-disordered breathing in African-Americans and Caucasians. Am J Respir Crit Care Med. 1997;155:186.
8. Epstein LJ, Kristo D, Strollo PJ Jr, et al. Clinical guideline for the evaluation, management and long-term care of obstructive sleep apnea in adults. J Clin Sleep Med. 2009;5:263.
9. Chiu HY, Chen PY, Chuang LP, et al. Diagnostic accuracy of the Berlin questionnaire, STOP-BANG, STOP, and Epworth sleepiness scale in detecting obstructive sleep apnea: a bivariate meta-analysis. Sleep Med Rev. 2017;36:57.
10. George CF. Sleep apnea, alertness, and motor vehicle crashes. Am J Respir Crit Care Med. 2007;176:954.
11. Chen YH, Keller JK, Kang JH, et al. Obstructive sleep apnea and the subsequent risk of depressive disorder: a population-based follow-up study. J Clin Sleep Med. 2013;9:417.
12. Peppard PE, Szklo-Coxe M, Kla KM, Young T. Longitudinal association of sleep-related breathing disorder and depression. Arch Intern Med. 2006;166:1709.
13. Botros N, Concato J, Mohsenin V, et al. Obstructive sleep apnea as a risk factor for type 2 diabetes. Am J Med. 2009;122:1122.
14. Punjabi NM, Shahar E, Redline S, et al. Sleep-disordered breathing, glucose intolerance, and insulin resistance: the sleep heart health study. Am J Epidemiol. 2004;160:521.
15. Turnbull F, Blood Pressure Lowering Treatment Trialists' Collaboration. Effects of different blood-pressure-lowering regimens on major cardiovascular events: results of prospectively-designed overviews of randomized trials. Lancet. 2003;362:1527.

16. Guilleminault C, Connolly SJ, Winkle RA. Cardiac arrhythmia and conduction disturbances during sleep in 400 patients with sleep apnea syndrome. Am J Cardiol. 1983;52:490.
17. Foster GD, Sanders MH, Millman R, et al. Obstructive sleep apnea among obese patients with type 2 diabetes. Diabetes Care. 2009;32:1017–9.
18. Abdelsattar ZM, Hendren S, Wong SL, et al. The impact of untreated obstructive sleep apnea on cardiopulmonary complications in general and vascular surgery: a cohort study. Sleep. 2015;38:1205.
19. Mokhlesi B, Hovda MD, Vekhter B, et al. Sleep disordered breathing and postoperative outcomes after elective surgery: analysis of the nationwide inpatient sample. Chest. 2013;144:903.
20. Kaw R, Chung F, Pasupuleti V, et al. Meta-analysis of the association between obstructive sleep apnoea and postoperative outcome. Br J Anaesth. 2012;109:897.
21. Punjabi NM, Caffo BS, Goodwin JL, et al. Sleep-disordered breathing and mortality: a prospective cohort study. PLoS Med. 2009;6:e1000132.
22. Marshall NS, Wong KK, Liu PY, et al. Sleep apnea as an independent risk factor for all-cause mortality: the Busselton health study. Sleep. 2008;31:1079.
23. Rosen CL, Auckley D, Benca R, et al. A multisite randomized trial of portable sleep studies and positive airway pressure autotitration versus laboratory-based polysomnography for the diagnosis and treatment of obstructive sleep apnea: the HomePAP study. Sleep. 2012;35:757–67.
24. Kapur VK, Auckley DH, Chowdhuri S, et al. Clinical practice guideline for diagnostic testing for adult obstructive sleep apnea: an American Academy of Sleep Medicine clinical practice guideline. J Clin Sleep Med. 2017;13:479.

Medical Management of Obstructive Sleep Apnea

2

William Taylor Palfrey, Peter Staiano, Kevin Green, Ashleigh Weyh, Salam O. Salman, and Mariam Louis

2.1 Positive Airway Pressure Therapy

2.1.1 Introduction

First-line therapy for most adult patients with obstructive sleep apnea (OSA) is positive airway pressure (PAP) applied via facial or nasal mask during hours of sleep. The application of PAP leads to a positive pharyngeal transmural pressure so that the intraluminal pressure overcomes the tendency of the airway to collapse and may stabilize the airway by increasing end-expiratory lung volumes leading a form of caudal traction [1]. By maintaining a patent airway, PAP is capable of reducing apneas and hypopneas [2] and increasing the average hemoglobin oxygenation while the patient is asleep [3]. It has been demonstrated to improve sleep quality and reduce symptoms of obstructive sleep apnea including daytime sleepiness, daytime neurocognitive performance, and snoring [3]. PAP has also been demonstrated to

W. T. Palfrey
Pulmonary Disease and Critical Care Medicine, Department of Medicine, College of Medicine, University of Florida—Jacksonville, Jacksonville, FL, USA
e-mail: william.palfrey@jax.ufl.edu

P. Staiano · K. Green
Internal Medicine, Department of Medicine, College of Medicine, University of Florida—Jacksonville, Jacksonville, FL, USA
e-mail: peter.staiano@jax.ufl.edu; kevin.green@jax.ufl.edu

A. Weyh · S. O. Salman
Department of Oral and Maxillofacial Surgery, College of Medicine, University of Florida—Jacksonville, Jacksonville, FL, USA
e-mail: salam.salman@jax.ufl.edu; ashleigh.weyh@jax.ufl.edu

M. Louis (✉)
Division of Pulmonary, Critical Care and Sleep Medicine, Department of Medicine, College of Medicine, University of Florida—Jacksonville, Jacksonville, FL, USA
e-mail: mariam.louis@jax.ufl.edu

S. O. Salman (ed.), *Modern Management of Obstructive Sleep Apnea*,
https://doi.org/10.1007/978-3-030-11443-5_2

improve outcomes of comorbidities related to the development and progression of OSA, including hypertension [4], metabolic derangements [5], and motor vehicle collisions [6]. This has been verified in various studies that examined the application of continuous positive airway pressure versus sham therapy.

Positive airway pressure has been recommended by the American Academy of Sleep Medicine (AASM) for all patients diagnosed with OSA [7], as defined by the respiratory disturbance index (RDI) and presence of any of the symptoms associated with obstructive sleep apnea syndrome (OSAS), such as sleepiness, nonrestorative sleep, arousal due to snoring, gasping, or choking, etc. In the United States, reimbursement from the Centers for Medicare and Medicaid Services (CMS) to cover PAP is based on the severity of the RDI and the presence of any symptoms or sequelae.

There are different types of PAP that can be used in the treatment of OSA. The most commonly prescribed is a fixed continuous positive airway pressure, (CPAP), which provides a set pressure throughout the entirety of the respiratory cycle. However, CPAP is not the only positive airway pressure modality that has been used to treat OSA. Bilevel positive airway pressure, or BPAP, is another modality that can be prescribed. BPAP utilizes one pressure setting for the expiratory phase of the respiratory cycle—EPAP—and a second pressure setting for the inspiratory phase—IPAP. BPAP is often utilized in patients who fail CPAP therapy; these patients continue to have symptoms or an unacceptably high apnea-hypopnea index (AHI), the number of apneas and hypopneas found per hour of testing. It is also often prescribed for those who have coexisting OSA and diseases that cause chronic hypercapnic respiratory failure, such as chronic obstructive pulmonary disease (COPD), obesity hypoventilation syndrome (OHS), chronic opioid use, or neuromuscular disorders that affect ventilation. Additionally, patients that have a combination of OSA along with central sleep apnea (CSA) may respond to BPAP. Finally, auto-titrating positive airway pressure, or APAP, is a form of PAP in which the device can detect obstructive events throughout the night and modify the PAP setting periodically to reduce the frequency of those events. It has been proposed for use in the following situations: patients who complain of intolerance of the dose of PAP pressure that is necessary to prevent events in all sleep positions and stages; patients who are subjected to factors that can vary their pressure requirement, like nasal congestion from allergies or frequent upper respiratory infections; or if access to CPAP titration study is limited or delayed. More advanced modalities such as BPAP with ST or adaptive servo-ventilation (ASV) are often used in the setting of more complex disease states such as the combination of OSA and heart failure.

The initiation of CPAP therapy is often directed by CPAP titration studies. These tests are performed following sleep studies that confirm the diagnosis of OSA. During the studies, continuous positive airway pressure is started at a low level for patient comfort—often 5 cm H_2O or less—and then slowly titrated up while electroencephalographic, pulse oximetry data, and patient positioning are recorded throughout the test. Optimal pressure dosage that provides for rapid eye movement (REM) sleep while in the supine position, as well as adequate oxyhemoglobin saturation, is then recommended by a certified sleep physician and ordered by the same sleep physician or the patient's other providers. Recommendations are often made at the same time regarding appropriate masks to use and whether to include heat and/or humidity to the circuit or a ramp of the pressure level.

Contraindications to long-term use of positive airway pressure include upper airway obstruction not related to a patient's functional upper airway obstruction, inability to cooperate with the therapy or protect their airway, inability to clear secretions, patients with facial trauma or deformity, or patients who are high risk for aspiration.

2.1.2 Compliance

Compliance, commonly defined as usage of >4 h/night with PAP therapy, is often the greatest initial hurdle to patients receiving the maximum benefit of therapy. It is estimated that 29–83% of patients are non-adherent to PAP. Studies suggest that >6 h/night of PAP usage results in normal levels of objectively measured and self-reported daytime sleepiness. Patients that have positions of employment in which daytime attention and neurocognitive performance is critical—truck drivers, air traffic controllers, etc.—may need more than the minimum 4 h of use nightly that is customarily considered to be compliant [8].

Several studies have shown that the initial experience with CPAP appears to be important predictor of compliance. As such, it is recommended that early evaluation of compliance be performed following the initiation of all PAP therapy. Ideally, patients should be re-evaluated within the first few weeks of therapy [9]. Compliance checks can be performed by requiring that the patient bring in to the office the data storage that is recorded from the CPAP machine, or for those machines equipped with modem or wireless technology, compliance can be checked remotely. Other predictors of compliance are self-reported daytime sleepiness (as measured by the Epworth Sleepiness Scale (ESS) of >10), greater severity of oxyhemoglobin desaturations during sleep, CPAP titration via an attended polysomnography, effect of CPAP on bed partner, and a motivated patient.

Several factors have been shown to predict nonadherence with PAP therapy: those related to the patient, those related to therapy and medication, and those related to the health professional prescribing the PAP. Patient-related factors include failure to understand the importance of or instructions concerning the therapy; physical limitations such as vision, hearing, or hand coordination; feeling too ill or tired to use the therapy; social isolation and lack of social support; and concomitant self-administration of additional medications or alcohol. Therapy- and medication-related factors include complexity or therapy or dosing, lack of efficacy, expense of the therapy, adverse reactions to therapy, and characteristics of the illness. Provider-related factors include poor provider-patient relationship, unwillingness to educate the patient, doubt concerning therapeutic potential, and lack of knowledge of medications that the patient is taking or has access to.

Several interventions can be applied to increase adherence. Compliance is jeopardized by the side effects associated with positive airway pressure therapy. It is recommended that the patient be offered a variety of masks prior to undergoing CPAP titration studies so that the optimum pressure dose using a comfortable mask may be ascertained and so that adherence to therapy can be encouraged. Nasal congestion may be alleviated with the use of adding heated humidity to the circuit during CPAP use. Air leaks and ingestion of air during use may be mitigated with the use of a chin strap. Aerophagia may also be addressed with the use of alternative positive airway pressure modalities, such as APAP. Cognitive behavioral therapy (CBT) has been used shortly following initiation of therapy to improve the likelihood of adherence. Overall, education about the potential side effects that may develop, and early and frequent follow-up after the initiation of CPAP therapy, is important to ensure that patients are receiving the maximum benefit of this treatment. It should be noted that the choice of PAP modality does not alter compliance. In addition, there is a paucity of data on the routine use of sedative-hypnotics at the time of CPAP initiation, and they should not be routinely used to potentially increase CPAP compliance.

2.1.3 Benefits

There have been a host of attempts made to improve compliance with CPAP therapy. Quick response to the development of side effects of CPAP can promote adherence to use. Though proper mask fitting is important, a 2018 study demonstrated that offering patients the chance to change their masks after the first compliance check does not improve compliance [10].

With all that is involved in diagnosing and treating obstructive sleep apnea, including multiple overnight stays in the sleep lab; durable medical equipment that must be ordered, fitted to the patient, and then carefully titrated in order to optimize the patient's response; and high failure rates, a question should be raised: What benefit does the patient receive for having jumped these hurdles and participated in the utilization of a therapy that is costly and cumbersome?

Treatment of OSA has been shown to improve blood pressure modestly, as already mentioned and can augment the use of antihypertensives in patients with both OSA and essential hypertension. CPAP can modify the risk of recurrent atrial fibrillation [11] and nocturnal ischemic cardiovascular events [12]. For patients with comorbid heart failure and OSA, the use of CPAP was associated with improvement in left ventricular ejection fraction [13]. The VAMONOS study showed that outstanding compliance to CPAP reduced fasting blood glucose in patients with OSA, and this may prove beneficial at reducing the rates of the development of diabetes mellitus in patients with OSA [14]. CPAP use has been shown to improve symptoms of depression as evidenced by lower PHQ-9 scores in those patients who were compliant with CPAP therapy [15]. These benefits are all in addition to the improvement in daytime sleepiness, snoring, and sleep quality already mentioned. In conclusion, while PAP therapy can be challenging, it still remains first-line treatment.

2.2 Positional and Medication Therapy

2.2.1 Introduction

Positional therapy is another treatment option in the management of OSA. The most important risk factor for OSA is obesity. Neck circumference increases with obesity as deposited adipose tissue increases the thickness of the lateral pharyngeal walls, leading to narrowing the airway. Sleeping in the supine position further exacerbates this process due to gravity drawing soft tissue into the pharyngeal space, further constricting the upper airway. Confounding risk factors include short mandibular size, tonsillar and adenoid hypertrophy, and a small midface. Cumulatively, this leads to increased upper airway resistance and decreased ventilation due to diminished neural output to the upper airway dilator muscles, chest wall, and accessory muscles. The current theory is that OSA is a progressive disease that may not be reversible if left untreated. A way to counter this pathophysiology is a method for the patient to sleep in the lateral recumbent position, called positional therapy.

There are various devices used in positional therapy; the classic example is a wedge-shaped device that restricts the patient from transitioning into a supine sleeping position. There are various other devices patients wear on the back which also function as a deterrent to sleeping in the supine position. Examples include wearing a T-shirt with a tennis ball attached to the back, a backpack with tennis balls or baseballs, or any other mechanism that will cause discomfort when lying supine. The rationale behind positional therapy is that the awkwardness will wake the patient, forcing them to sleep in the lateral recumbent position. In one study comparing sleep positional therapy and tennis ball method in positional OSA, success was achieved in improving respiratory indices [16]. The goal of AHI <5 was achieved in 68% of sleep positional therapy patients and 42.9% of those using the tennis ball technique. However, sleep positional therapy was shown to significantly outperform tennis ball technique in the categories of compliance, quality of life, and sleep quality compared to the tennis ball technique. Tennis ball technique can be a cheap option if patients elect to make their own positional therapy device, such as wearing a backpack with a baseball inside. However, this may be cumbersome, and compliance with these devices is typically low.

There are newer, more compact sleep positional therapy devices which show promise. Three have so far been approved by the US Food and Drug Agency (FDA). These include the Zzoma Device (a light semirigid wedge-shaped device that is attached to the upper torso), the Night Shift Sleep Positioner (a battery powered neck-positioning device), and the SONA Pillow (a double incline triangular pillow). Other devices are available on the market but are not FDA approved. These include the chest vibratory device that sends impulses until the patient changes to a nonsupine position [17, 18], as well as the Rematee Bumper Belt [19].

Numerous studies have investigated the efficacy of positional therapy. When compared to nonstandard therapy, positional therapy led to significant reductions in AHI, time spent in the supine position, as well as reductions in ODI [20, 21]. When compared to CPAP therapy, CPAP therapy was more effective at reducing AHI compared to positional therapy [22, 23]. A recent study published in *Journal of Sleep Medicine* in 2017 [24] evaluated the newer positional therapy devices as described above. The study demonstrated improvement in AHI by 54%, and had a high compliance rate with a median rate of 92.7–96%, at 1 month follow-up. However, the vast majority of studies are small case series and cohort studies. Large good-quality randomized controlled trials with long-term follow-up are lacking. This poses a limitation in providing a good evidence base for the routine use of PT in clinical practice. In addition, outcome measurements have focused primarily on AHI. There are a few studies looking at secondary outcomes such as sleepiness and quality of life measurements, and measuring compliance remains a challenge.

Given the lack of robust clinical trials, this treatment modality is most appropriate for positional OSA patients with a non-supine apnea-hypopnea index (AHI) < 5 or OSA patients who have a non-supine AHI less than the overall AHI. It can also be used as salvage therapy in patients who cannot tolerate CPAP. However, positional therapy is not effective for patients who have non-positional sleep apnea, as their sleeping derangements are not affected by body position.

Additional studies are needed looking at long-term compliance and to further evaluate positional therapy as both a primary and adjunct treatment modality for positional obstructive sleep apnea.

2.2.2 Medications for the Treatment of OSA

Currently, there are no proven effective medication options available for the treatment of OSA.

Various medications have been studied; however none were shown to be of statistically significant value [25]. Examples of previously studied medications include but are not limited to progesterone, fluticasone, mirtazapine, physostigmine, donepezil, and paroxetine among many others. A study published in 2013 [25] performed a meta-analysis of 30 trials that studied 25 medications including the ones mentioned previously. It was concluded that none of the medications studied showed sufficient evidence to recommend their use. Interestingly, a new study published in 2018 [26] which investigated hypertension and OSA compared acetazolamide combined with CPAP to acetazolamide and CPAP individually. The acetazolamide alone and acetazolamide combined with CPAP arms were both shown to decrease mean arterial blood pressure by 7 mmHg. Additionally, the AHI was significantly reduced in all three arms, the most significant being the combined acetazolamide and CPAP arm. However, this study was very small (only 13 subjects enrolled) and was only investigated for 2-week periods. Additional larger-scale studies will be needed to confirm the efficacy of acetazolamide in OSA management.

Cannabinoids have been investigated more recently as a potential treatment option. However, a recent article suggests that cannabinoids may improve in sleep disordered breathing. Thus far, these investigations have been met with mixed results. There currently is a promising phase II trial investigating the effects of the medication Dronabinol, a synthetic version of delta-9 tetrahydrocannabinol (THC) [27].

This medication is currently FDA approved but only for the treatment of nausea and vomiting in patients receiving chemotherapy. According to a recent article published in Sleep Journal in 2018, results so far demonstrated that patients with moderate-severe OSA had a significant reduction in AHI, as well as subjective improvement in their sleepiness with Dronabinol, when compared to placebo. One hypothesis is that OSA patients may benefit from cannabinoids due to their effects on serotonin-related apneic episodes.

The role of Dronabinol in treatment of OSA has yet to be determined; however, the data so far suggests it may be an option for patients in the future who fail CPAP or require an adjunct to their current regimen. While sleep latency appears to be improved with Dronabinol, one study suggests that there may be some concern that Dronabinol could have a long-term negative effect on sleep quality [28]. Additional long-term studies, including a phase 3 trial, will need to be performed before this medication is a viable option in the OSA population. In conclusion, there are currently no recommendations for the use of medications in the treatment of OSA.

2.3 Weight Loss

2.3.1 Introduction

Obesity is the strongest risk factor for the development of OSA and also plays a role in disease progression. Although a modifiable independent risk factor is treatable, many patients solely rely on continuous positive airway pressure (CPAP) without addressing weight management. The prevalence of obesity in adults in the United States is estimated at 39.8%, which has increased by over 3% in the past 2 years [29, 30].

Obesity, particularly visceral obesity, exhibits mechanical, neurochemical, and anatomical alterations that predispose individuals to upper airway obstruction while sleeping. Obesity contributes to reductions in lung volumes and increasing pharyngeal collapsibility. Adipose deposition around the neck increases the neck circumference and contributes to airway narrowing. In addition, the presence of adipokines (central nervous system signaling proteins) has a detrimental effect on neuromuscular control, which ultimately influences upper airway collapsibility and sleep apnea severity [31]. Interestingly, weight loss reduces upper airway collapsibility during sleep; however whether this is primarily due to alterations in mechanical and anatomical properties, or due to improved neuromuscular control, is controversial, as weight loss does improve hyperlipidemia, leptin levels, and insulin resistance [32, 33].

Whatever the mechanism by which weight loss improves OSA, weight loss is a highly effective strategy for management of sleep apnea. A ten to fifteen percent decrease in total body weight has been proven to decrease the sleep apnea severity index by up to 50% in obese male patients [34, 35]. Although the process of weight loss can be challenging, especially in those where mobility is limited by obesity, the results of weight loss are well established as a disease modifying agent and can be a curative intervention as well. Weight loss discussion should include an interdisciplinary approach including primary care physicians, pulmonologists, and dieticians, among others with a common goal of weight loss while improving patient satisfaction. Although weight loss is effective, it is not always curative as many do not achieve ideal BMI. However, it can only help to augment OSA therapy and minimize severity.

Weight loss options for OSA are classified into medical and surgical approaches each with their own caveats.

2.3.2 Medical Weight Loss

Medical weight loss include lifestyle changes, exercise, diet, medications (orlistat, fluoxetine, phentermine), and cognitive behavioral therapy. The risks and complications of medical therapy are far less than surgical interventions; however the pace and degree of weight loss are usually significantly lower. Although weight loss is mentioned in the clinical guidelines, there is a paucity of well-executed studies discerning the impact lifestyle interventions have on OSA. Meta-analysis of randomized control trials involving the effects of lifestyle intervention (low-calorie diet, liquid meals replacements, diet and exercise information, and behavioral therapy) showed that a weight reduction of 14 kilograms resulted in a decrease in AHI by 16 events per hour. In clinical trials only, a minority of patients have been cured with medical weight loss. Medical weight loss is often sluggish and time-consuming and requires close follow-up with multiple specialists (physicians, dietitians, and personal trainers) which can ultimately lead to lack of adherence.

2.3.3 Surgical Weight Loss

Surgical intervention is a complex decision involving the patient's comorbidities, psychiatric assessment, and previous attempts at healthy weight loss. After an ample trial of a multidisciplinary approach to weight loss, bariatric surgery is considered for patients who have a BMI > 35 kg/m^2 with the presence of obesity-related comorbidities (type II diabetes, hypertension, sleep apnea, and others) or BMI > 40 kg/m^2 without any complications. Bariatric surgery promotes weight loss by caloric restriction, malabsorption, or both. The data comparing efficacy of the distinct types (Roux-en-Y gastric bypass, laparoscopic sleeve gastrectomy, and biliopancreatic diversion of bariatric procedures) in the management of OSA are sparse. However, the impact of bariatric surgery in OSA population has resulted in higher cure and improvement rates than medical weight loss groups, likely due to the dramatic sustained weight loss seen after surgical intervention. Over 80% of patients who undergo bariatric surgery will see improvement or resolution of OSA symptoms. In a small minority of patients, bariatric weight loss may result in cessation of upper airway collapsibility; however, many patients may equate their improvement in their symptoms as a cure. Inappropriate termination of CPAP use may lead to increased cardiovascular risks and weight gain. Although beneficial, surgical intervention is not without risk. Complications include steatorrhea, iron deficiency, and fat-soluble vitamin deficiencies [36–38].

2.3.4 Weight Loss in Combination with CPAP

Regardless of the manner chosen to achieve weight loss, patients using CPAP in combination with weight loss require close follow-up to ensure continued adherence with all aspects of therapy. For many patients, liberation from CPAP is a major motivation for weight loss; however CPAP adherence decreases as a result. Reductions in compliance are likely due to an assortment of factors including unfavorable CPAP titration, improvement in symptoms, and changes in facial fat area resulting in improper mask fitting. Indeed, there is a linear relationship between visceral fat loss and midfacial fat volume loss; whereby alterations in the facial structure following significant weight loss can lead to air leakage, rendering the CPAP system unusable [38–40]. After significant weight loss, physicians should subsequently ensure proper consideration is made regarding proper mask fitting, pressure requirements, and continued CPAP adherence if necessary. Significant weight changes have been proven to reduce the mean optimal CPAP pressure by approximately 3 cm H_2O.

Weight loss with CPAP use should be encouraged. A randomized control trial sought to examine the relationship between C-reactive protein (CRP) levels in OSA patients being treated with CPAP alone vs CPAP combined with weight loss treatment. CRP levels were used as a marker of cardiovascular disease. In the groups treated with combined CPAP and weight loss, the CRP levels declined significantly more than those treated with CPAP alone. Combination therapy also showed reduction in hyperlipidemia, hypertension, blood pressure, and insulin sensitivity [32, 33, 41]. As seen in the Sleep Apnea Cardiovascular Endpoints (SAVE) study, CPAP therapy alone did not prevent cardiovascular events in patients with known cardiovascular disease and moderate-to-severe OSA [42]. However, the patients enrolled in the SAVE study only used CPAP for 3.3 h/night, well below what is considered to be compliant. The combination of these studies highlights the importance of accompanying a weight loss treatment strategy along with CPAP therapy in obese patients with OSA.

2.3.5 Weight Loss and Exercise

Weight loss and exercise should be recommended to all patients with OSA who are overweight or obese. While rarely leading to complete remission of OSA, weight loss, including that from bariatric surgery, and exercise have been shown to improve overall health and metabolic parameters. They can also decrease the apnea-hypopnea index (AHI), reduce blood pressure, improve quality of life, and likely decrease excessive daytime somnolence.

2.4 Oral Appliance Therapy

2.4.1 Introduction

Oral appliances (OAs) have been used in the treatment of obstructive sleep apnea (OSA) since the 1980s. It was then that Cartwright and Samelson first published about a nonsurgical treatment for OSA, with a tongue-retaining device. Since that time, there have been many different appliance designs, with over 100 currently on the market, and many more to likely emerge in the future. OAs currently are the second most common treatment of OSA. They are recommended for patients with mild-to-moderate OSA and, for severe cases, only when patients are unable to tolerate CPAP [43]. Multiple studies have shown patients generally prefer OAs over CPAP and have better reported compliance [44]. A multidisciplinary team approach to treatment is vital for maximizing treatment outcomes. Teams should involve a sleep physician, dentist, sleep surgeon to evaluate for source of obstruction, and a general medicine physician. Additionally, all patients, regardless of OSA severity, should first be counseled on lifestyle changes, including weight loss and cessation of alcohol use.

2.4.2 Patient Selection

Patients should not be seen for fabrication of an OA without a referral from a trained sleep medicine physician, who performed a full evaluation of the patient. If nasal obstruction is suspected as the etiology of the OSA, the patient should be referred to sleep surgeon for evaluation. Nasal obstruction can cause increased mouth breathing, which decreases hypopharyngeal space and increases upper airway resistance, leading to more apneas and hypopneas [45]. All patients will need a comprehensive oral examination, including evaluation of the dentition, temporomandibular joints (TMJ), and supporting tissues prior to fabrication of an OA. Patients should not have active decay or periodontitis, as an OA can exacerbate both. A stable dentition is needed, with ideally at minimum ten teeth per arch; however some authors have recommended as few as six [46], distributed evenly among the arches. Included in the comprehensive oral exam is obtaining radiographic images, specifically, a lateral cephalogram and panoramic radiograph. These images are important for the evaluation of the patients' dentition and skeletal relationship and also serve as a baseline prior to initiating OA therapy. Patients with bruxism should be identified at this stage, as they will be at higher risk of breaking an OA not made of durable materials. TMJ evaluation should reveal unrestricted lateral, vertical, and protrusive excursive movements and a healthy, pain-free TMJ complex. OAs can exacerbate pain if there is restriction, causing patients to be less compliant with treatment. Lastly, patients need to have a current diagnosis of mild or moderate OSA with polysomnography (PSG) and a desire for nonsurgical treatment. CPAP is almost always offered as the first-line treatment, so referred patients are likely known to be refractory to CPAP.

2.4.3 Mechanism of Oral Appliances

Common features shared by OSA patients are mandibular retrognathism, retropositioning of the tongue, inferior positioned hyoid bone, tonsillar hypertrophy, or nasal obstruction [46]. OAs are able to overcome retrognathism and retropositioning of the tongue by functioning to protrude the mandible or tongue with the purpose of increasing the upper airway volume and reducing pharyngeal collapsibility [47]. There are multiple etiologies for OSA, so OAs will therefore have a variable treatment outcome for different patients. OAs can effectively improve pharyngeal collapsibility; however they have no effect on patients with overly sensitive ventilatory control systems or reduced arousal thresholds [48]. Titratable devices are the most common and effective and are recommended by the author. They are constructed as an upper and lower part, with intermaxillary adjustment mechanism between them allowing for forward movement of the mandible into optimal position [49]. OAs that allow for mouth opening are less effective in reducing OSA [50]. The use of non-custom-made devices is also not recommended, due to inferior fit and retention, which could affect overall patient comfort and compliance.

2.4.4 Types of Oral Appliances

There are two classifications of OAs for OSA: (1) mandibular repositioning devices (MRDs) and (2) tongue-retainer devices (TRDs). MRDs have the ability to position the mandible and tongue forward anywhere from 50 to 100% of maximum protrusive movement as tolerated, therefore brining attached soft tissue anteriorly and opening the pharyngeal airway (Fig. 2.1). MRDs have better reported compliance than TRDs and are more widely used [51]. TRDs protract the tongue into a bulb compartment on the device, through use of negative pressure. They do not need support from the teeth, which makes them ideal for patients with an insufficient number teeth or poor distribution, as well as periodontitis.

2.4.5 Fabrication and Delivery

The authors prefer and recommend the use of custom oral appliances. This requires obtaining impressions of the maxillary and mandibular arches, as well as a bite registration in centric occlusion. The impressions, and/or dental casts, and bite registration are then sent to a dental lab to fabricate the prosthesis. Once patients are fitted with their OA, they should titrate to effect. Patients will need to be seen for adjustments after delivery, usually only for 3 months. During this period the patient will work with just the dentist or other practitioner to titrate the OA to ideal therapeutic position. At 6 months, patients should return to their sleep medicine physician for repeat PSG to evaluate response to treatment. Once treatment goals with the OA are met, the patient should be seen by their practitioner every 6 months for the first 2 years, then annually. At these visits, patients should be evaluated for

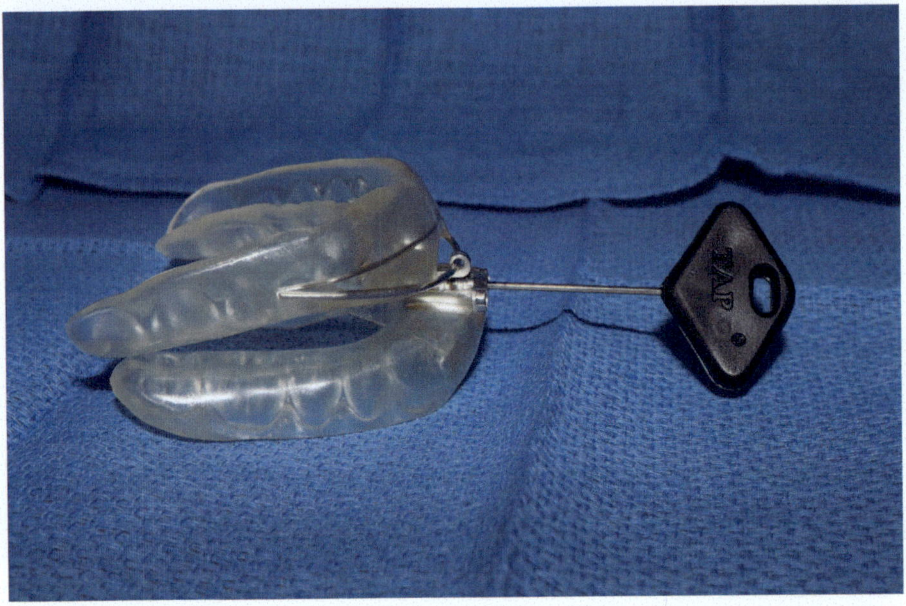

Fig. 2.1 DreamTap picture

subjective symptoms of snoring and sleepiness via the Epworth Sleepiness Scale (ESS), assessed for changes in the integrity of the OA, and monitored for side effects. Annual radiographic (i.e., panorex/lateral cephalogram or CBCT) images should be obtained as well, to evaluate for any changes in dentition and occlusion. If there is any evidence that the OA is no longer effective, the patient should be referred back to the sleep physician. OAs can last 5 or more years but may need periodic adjustments.

2.4.6 Outcomes

Studies have shown OAs are able to reduce AHI and ESS scores and on average reduce the RDI by 56% [49, 52]. They can also be as effective as CPAP in patients with positional OSA [53]. Treatment success across all levels of OSA severity with OAs is approximately 50%, with average reduction in baseline AHI of 55%. They also have been shown to have positive effects on snoring and daytime sleepiness, but less so than CPAP, and can increase quality of life. A recent meta-analysis showed treatment successes were less in severe OSA, but 70% of patients still had reduction in AHI greater than or equal to 50%, while 23% had complete resolution of OSA [54]. Of note, better results have been found with custom-made OAs compared to prefabricated devices [55]. Additionally, younger, nonobese females have been found to have greater success with OAs, and those who gained weight during treatment had a positive correlation with treatment failure [56].

Because patients have the ability to self-titrate, there will be a difference in outcomes based on variability in movement of the lower jaw forward. Success of an OA positively correlates with a less collapsible upper airway and less sensitive ventilatory control system [57]. Patients can be screened prior to fabrication of OA with nasoendoscopy to see if they are a good candidate based on their airway anatomy [58]. Once OAs are delivered, some practitioners administer type 3 or 4 home sleep tests to assess the need for changes in titration. This can be useful in patients that never experienced subjective symptoms, such as snoring or daytime sleepiness. These sleep tests are not diagnostic but are solely to aid with adjustments to the OA.

2.4.7 Side Effects

Reported side effects of oral appliances included excessive salivation, mouth or tooth discomfort, occlusal change, pain in teeth, muscle stiffness, and symptoms of temporomandibular joint disorder. Custom OAs can be designed and adjusted to reduce pressure on the teeth and gums. The most frequent cause of poor compliance with OAs is discomfort. However, most of these side effects only last for the first few months of use [49]. Morning jaw exercises have been shown to improve compliance, reduce most of the side effects, as well as aid the mandible into returning to its normal position [59]. There are also morning repositioning devices available that patients wear for 20 min to assist with stretching after removing their OA [46]. Of note, one study also found patients taking statins experienced more myofascial pain initially with OA therapy [60].

Due to the anterior forces on the mandibular teeth, and the distal forces on the maxillary teeth, most patients can expect decrease in overbite and overjet during the first 5 years of treatment. Bite changes will continue to progress as long as treatment is continued, with median changes in overbite of −1.6 mm and −1.1 mm change to overjet after a 17-year period [61]. However, a majority of patients report they don't notice the change, likely because there is no loss of posterior occlusion or associated TMD [62]. Periodic re-evaluation will be needed because this forward movement of mandibular teeth can result in the device to produce less mandibular advancement and less treatment efficacy over time. Studies show that most patients need further titration over time to compensate for tooth movement [61].

2.4.8 Oral Appliances vs Continuous Positive Airway Pressure

Current first-line therapies for OSA include continuous positive airway pressure (CPAP), OAs, and modified sleep positioning. CPAP is frequently employed before OAs, but the adherence to this therapy is problematic. Overall acceptance rate is approximately 50%, and it has been found that true compliance is much lower than patient reported compliance [52]. Still, the variability in treatment response among patients to OAs makes CPAP currently the most efficient therapy option. This is because even though OAs have proven to be effective, they are still less predictable than CPAP.

OAs can be used in combination with CPAP, either wearing both at the same time or alternating modalities nightly. Combination therapy has been proven effective for patients who cannot tolerate both OAs and CPAP, because patients can do less advancement with the OA and use lower pressures with CPAP, making the therapies more tolerable [63]. OAs can also be used as an adjunct in patients with partial success on CPAP or with positional therapy [63, 64].

2.4.9 Conclusion

OAs are indicated for the management of patients with mild-to-moderate severity OSA and can be considered in patients with severe OSA that are unable to tolerate CPAP. There are numerous OAs available on the market, all varying slightly in design; however there is no identified gold standard device to date. After referral from a sleep medicine physician, PSG, and through oral examination, it is recommended to fabricate a custom, adjustable, and titratable mandibular repositioning device, such as the dreamTAP™ (Airway Management, Carrollton, TX). Prefabricated devices are not recommended by the authors. Once the OA is fabricated and delivered, patients should use them nightly and titrate to effect. A repeat PSG can be conducted at 6 months. With prolonged use of OAs, most patients experience some changes in occlusion; however they are minor and often not recognized by the patient. Long-term studies have shown OAs can successfully treat OSA, but it is expected OAs effectiveness can decline long term due to progression of disease and patient compliance.

References

1. Jordan AS, McSharry DG, Malhotra A. Adult obstructive sleep apnoea. Lancet. 2014;383(9918):736. Epub 2013 Aug 2.
2. Jonas DE, Amick HR, Feltner C, Weber RP, Arvanitis M, Stine A, Lux L, Harris RP. Screening for obstructive sleep apnea in adults: evidence report and systematic review for the US preventive services task force. JAMA. 2017;317(4):415.
3. Giles TL, Lesserson TJ, Smith BJ, White J, Wright J, Cates CJ. Continuous positive airways pressure for obstructive sleep apnoea in adults. Cochrane Database Syst Rev. 2006;(3):CD001106.
4. Martinez-Garcia MA, Capote F, Campos-Rodriguez F, et al. Effect of CPAP on blood pressure in patients with obstructive sleep apnea and resistant hypertension: the HIPARCO randomized clinical trial. JAMA. 2013;310(22):2407–15. https://doi.org/10.1001/jama.2013.281250.
5. Sharma SK, Agrawal S, Damodaran D, Sreenivas V, Kadhiravan T, Lakshmy R, Jagia P, Kumar A. CPAP for the metabolic syndrome in patients with obstructive sleep apnea. N Engl J Med. 2011;365(24):2277–86. https://doi.org/10.1056/NEJMoa1103944.
6. George CF. Reduction in motor vehicle collisions following treatment of sleep apnoea with nasal CPAP. Thorax. 2001;56(7):508–12.
7. Epstein LJ, Kristo D, Strollo PJ Jr, et al., for the Adult Obstructive Sleep Apnea Task Force of the American Academy of Sleep Medicine. Clinical guideline for the evaluation, management and long-term care of obstructive sleep apnea in adults. J Clin Sleep Med. 2009;5(3):263.

8. Weaver TE, Maislin G, Dinges DF, et al. Relationship between hours of CPAP use and achieving normal levels of sleepiness and daily functioning. Sleep. 2007;30(6):711–9.
9. Wolkove N, Baltzan M, Kamel H, et al. Long-term compliance with continuous positive airway pressure in patients with obstructive sleep apnea. Can Respir J. 2008;15(7):265–9.
10. Mastromatto N, Killough N, Keenan B, Schwab R, Bergmann A, Simonsen S, Staley B, Bae C, Schutte-Rodin S. 1075 the effect of changing the first CPAP mask on compliance. Sleep. 2018;41(Suppl_1):A399–400. https://doi.org/10.1093/sleep/zsy061.1074.
11. Shukla A, Aizer A, Holmes D, et al. Effect of obstructive sleep apnea treatment on atrial fibrillation recurrence. JACC Clin Electrophysiol. 2015;1(1–2):41–51. https://doi.org/10.1016/j.jacep.2015.02.014.
12. Peled N, Abinader EG, Pillar G, et al. Nocturnal ischemic events in patients with obstructive sleep apnea syndrome and ischemic heart disease: effects of continuous positive air pressure treatment. JACC. 1999;34(6):1744–9.
13. Kaneko Y, Floras JS, Usui K, et al. Cardiovascular effects of continuous positive airway pressure in patients with heart failure and obstructive sleep apnea. N Engl J Med. 2003;348(13):1233–41.
14. Ioachimescu OC, Anthony J Jr, Constantin T, et al. VAMONOS (Veterans Affairs' Metabolism, Obstructed and Non-Obstructed Sleep) study: effects of CPAP therapy on glucose metabolism in patients with obstructive sleep apnea. J Clin Sleep Med. 2017;13(3):455–66. https://doi.org/10.5664/jcsm.6502.
15. Edwards C, Mukherjee S, Simpson L, et al. Depressive symptoms before and after treatment of obstructive sleep apnea in men and women. J Clin Sleep Med. 2015;11(9):1029–38. https://doi.org/10.5664/jcsm.5020.
16. Eijsvogel MM, Ubbink R, Dekker J, Oppersma E, de Jongh FH, van der Palen J, Brusse-Keizer MG. Sleep position trainer versus tennis ball technique in positional obstructive sleep apnea syndrome. J Clin Sleep Med. 2015;11(2):139–47.
17. Bignold JJ, Mercer JD, Antic NA, McEvoy RD, Catcheside PG. Accurate position monitoring and improved supine-dependent obstructive sleep apnea with a new position recording and supine avoidance device. J Clin Sleep Med. 2011;7(4):376–83.
18. Levendowski DJ, Seagraves S, Popovic D, Westbrook PR. Assessment of a neck-based treatment and monitoring device for positional obstructive sleep apnea. J Clin Sleep Med. 2014;10(8):863–71.
19. Matthews L, Fortier N. The Rematee Bumper Belt® positional therapy device for snoring and obstructive sleep apnea: positional effectiveness in healthy subjects. Can J Respir Ther. 2013;49:11–4.
20. Cartwright R, et al. A comparative study of treatments for positional sleep apnea. Sleep. 1991;14:546–52.
21. Jackson M, et al. Efficacy of sleep position modification to treat positional obstructive sleep apnea. Sleep Med. 2015;16:545–52.
22. Skinner MA, et al. Efficacy of the 'tennis ball technique' versus nCPAP in the management of position-dependent obstructive sleep apnoea syndrome. Respirology. 2008;13:708–15.
23. Jokic R, et al. Positional treatment vs continuous positive airway pressure in patients with positional obstructive sleep apnea syndrome. Chest. 1999;115:771–81.
24. Ravesloot MJ, White D, Heinzer R, Oksenberg A, Pépin JL. Efficacy of the new generation of devices for positional therapy for patients with positional obstructive sleep apnea: a systematic review of the literature and meta-analysis. J Clin Sleep Med. 2017;13(6):813–24.
25. Mason M, Welsh EJ, Smith I. Drug therapy for obstructive sleep apnea in adults. Cochrane Database of Syst Rev. 2013;(5):CD003002. https://doi.org/10.1002/14651858.CD003002.pub3.
26. Eskandari D, Zou D, Grote L, Hoff E, Hedner J. Acetazolamide reduces blood pressure and sleep-disordered breathing in patients with hypertension and obstructive sleep apnea: a randomized controlled trial. J Clin Sleep Med. 2018;14(3):309–17.
27. Carley DW, Prasad B, Reid KJ, Malkani R, Attarian H, Abbott SM, Vern B, Xie H, Yuan C, Zee PC. Pharmacotherapy of apnea by cannabimimetic enhancement, the PACE clinical

trial: effects of dronabinol in obstructive sleep apnea. Sleep. 2018;41(1):zsx184. https://doi.org/10.1093/sleep/zsx184.
28. Babson KA, Sottile J, Morabito D. Cannabis, cannabinoids, and sleep: a review of the literature. Curr Psychiatry Rep. 2017;19:23.
29. Hales CM, Carroll MD, Fryar CD, Ogden CL. Prevalence of obesity among adults and youth: United States, 2015–2016. NCHS Data Brief. 2017;(288):1–8.
30. Ogden CL, Carroll MD, Fryar CD, Flegal KM. Prevalence of obesity among adults and youth: United States, 2011–2014. NCHS Data Brief. 2015;(219):1–8.
31. Schwartz AR, Patil SP, Laffan AM, Polotsky V, Schneider H, Smith PL. Obesity and obstructive sleep apnea: pathogenic mechanisms and therapeutic approaches. Proc Am Thorac Soc. 2008;5:185–92. https://doi.org/10.1513/pats.200708-137MG.
32. Romero-Corral A, Caples SM, Lopez-Jimenez F, Somers VK. Interactions between obesity and obstructive sleep apnea: implications for treatment. Chest. 2010;137:711–9. https://doi.org/10.1378/chest.09-0360.
33. Owens RL, Shafazand S. Effects of CPAP and weight loss on OSA outcomes. J Clin Sleep Med. 2014;10:1365–7. https://doi.org/10.5664/jcsm.4308.
34. Schwartz AR, Gold AR, Schubert N, Stryzak A, Wise RA, Permutt S, Smith PL. Effect of weight loss on upper airway collapsibility in obstructive sleep apnea. Am Rev Respir Dis. 1991;144:494–8. https://doi.org/10.1164/ajrccm/144.3_Pt_1.494.
35. Smith PL, Gold AR, Meyers DA, Haponik EF, Bleecker ER. Weight loss in mildly to moderately obese patients with obstructive sleep apnea. Ann Intern Med. 1985;103:850–5.
36. Sarkhosh K, Switzer NJ, El-Hadi M, Birch DW, Shi X, Karmali S. The impact of bariatric surgery on obstructive sleep apnea: a systematic review. Obes Surg. 2013;23:414–23. https://doi.org/10.1007/s11695-012-0862-2.
37. Priyadarshini P, Singh VP, Aggarwal S, Garg H, Sinha S, Guleria R. Impact of bariatric surgery on obstructive sleep apnoea-hypopnea syndrome in morbidly obese patients. J Minim Access Surg. 2017;13:291–5. https://doi.org/10.4103/jmas.JMAS_5_17.
38. Joosten SA, Hamilton GS, Naughton MT. Impact of weight loss management in OSA. Chest. 2017;152:194–203. https://doi.org/10.1016/j.chest.2017.01.027.
39. Lettieri CJ, Eliasson AH, Greenburg DL. Persistence of obstructive sleep apnea after surgical weight loss. J Clin Sleep Med. 2008;4:333–8.
40. Sawyer AM, Gooneratne NS, Marcus CL, Ofer D, Richards KC, Weaver TE. A systematic review of CPAP adherence across age groups: clinical and empiric insights for developing CPAP adherence interventions. Sleep Med Rev. 2011;15:343–56. https://doi.org/10.1016/j.smrv.2011.01.003.
41. Chirinos JA, Gurubhagavatula I, Teff K, Rader DJ, Wadden TA, Townsend R, Foster GD, Maislin G, Saif H, Broderick P, Chittams J, Hanlon AL, Pack AI. CPAP, weight loss, or both for obstructive sleep apnea. N Engl J Med. 2014;370:2265–75. https://doi.org/10.1056/NEJMoa1306187.
42. McEvoy RD, Antic NA, Heeley E, Luo Y, Ou Q, Zhang X, Mediano O, Chen R, Drager LF, Liu Z, Chen G, Du B, McArdle N, Mukherjee S, Tripathi M, Billot L, Li Q, Lorenzi-Filho G, Barbe F, Redline S, Wang J, Arima H, Neal B, White DP, Grunstein RR, Zhong N, Anderson CS. CPAP for prevention of cardiovascular events in obstructive sleep apnea. N Engl J Med. 2016;375:919–31. https://doi.org/10.1056/NEJMoa1606599.
43. Kushida CA, Morgenthaler TI, Littner MR, et al. Practice parameters for the treatment of snoring and obstructive sleep apnea with oral appliances: an update for 2005. Sleep. 2006;29(2):240–3. https://doi.org/10.1093/sleep/29.2.240.
44. Phillips CL, Grunstein RR, Darendeliler MA, et al. Health outcomes of continuous positive airway pressure versus oral appliance treatment for obstructive sleep apnea: a randomized controlled trial. Am J Respir Crit Care Med. 2013;187(8):879–87. https://doi.org/10.1164/rccm.201212-2223OC.
45. Fitzpatrick MF, McLean H, Urton AM, Tan A, O'Donnell D, Driver HS. Effect of nasal or oral breathing route on upper airway resistance during sleep. Eur Respir J. 2003;22(5):827–32. https://doi.org/10.1183/09031936.03.00047903.

46. Correa LP. Overview of oral appliance therapy for the management of obstructive sleep apnea. Sleep Med Clin. 2013;8(4):505–16. https://doi.org/10.1016/j.jsmc.2013.07.007.
47. Sutherland K, Chan ASL, Cistulli PA. Three-dimensional assessment of anatomical balance and oral appliance treatment outcome in obstructive sleep apnoea. Sleep Breath. 2016;20(3):903–10. https://doi.org/10.1007/s11325-015-1304-x.
48. Edwards BA, Eckert DJ, Jordan AS. Obstructive sleep apnoea pathogenesis from mild to severe: is it all the same? Respirology. 2017;22(1):33–42. https://doi.org/10.1111/resp.12913.
49. Marklund M. Update on oral appliance therapy for OSA. Curr Sleep Med Rep. 2017;3(3):143–51. https://doi.org/10.1007/s40675-017-0080-5.
50. Norrhem N, Marklund M. An oral appliance with or without elastic bands to control mouth opening during sleep—a randomized pilot study. Sleep Breath. 2016;20(3):929–38. https://doi.org/10.1007/s11325-016-1312-5.
51. Deane SA, Cistulli PA, Ng AT, Zeng B, Petocz P, Darendeliler MA. Comparison of mandibular advancement splint and tongue stabilizing device in obstructive sleep apnea: a randomized controlled trial. Sleep. 2009;32(5):648–53. https://doi.org/10.1093/sleep/32.5.648.
52. Bagheri SC. Clinical review of oral and maxillofacial surgery: a case-based approach. 2nd ed. St. Louis: Elsevier/Mosby; 2014. https://doi.org/10.1016/C2012-0-02809-8.
53. Takaesu Y, Tsuiki S, Kobayashi M, Komada Y, Nakayama H, Inoue Y. Mandibular advancement device as a comparable treatment to nasal continuous positive airway pressure for positional obstructive sleep apnea. J Clin Sleep Med. 2016;12(8):1113–9. https://doi.org/10.5664/jcsm.6048.
54. Sutherland K, Takaya H, Qian J, Petocz P, Ng AT, Cistulli PA. Oral appliance treatment response and polysomnographic phenotypes of obstructive sleep apnea. J Clin Sleep Med. 2015;11(8):861–8. https://doi.org/10.5664/jcsm.4934.
55. Serra-Torres S, Bellot-Arcís C, Montiel-Company JM, Marco-Algarra J, Almerich-Silla JM. Effectiveness of mandibular advancement appliances in treating obstructive sleep apnea syndrome: a systematic review. Laryngoscope. 2016;126(2):507–14. https://doi.org/10.1002/lary.25505.
56. Marklund M, Stenlund H, Franklin KA. Mandibular advancement devices in 630 men and women with obstructive sleep apnea and snoring: tolerability and predictors of treatment success. Chest. 2004;125(4):1270–8. https://doi.org/10.1378/chest.125.4.1270.
57. Edwards BA, Andara C, Landry S, et al. Upper-airway collapsibility and loop gain predict the response to oral appliance therapy in patients with obstructive sleep apnea. Am J Respir Crit Care Med. 2016;194(11):1413–22. https://doi.org/10.1164/rccm.201601-0099OC.
58. Sasao Y, Nohara K, Okuno K, Nakamura Y, Sakai T. Videoendoscopic diagnosis for predicting the response to oral appliance therapy in severe obstructive sleep apnea. Sleep Breath. 2014;18(4):809–15. https://doi.org/10.1007/s11325-014-0947-3.
59. Cunali PA, Almeida FR, Santos CD, et al. Mandibular exercises improve mandibular advancement device therapy for obstructive sleep apnea. Sleep Breath. 2011;15(4):717–27. https://doi.org/10.1007/s11325-010-0428-2.
60. González M, Macias-Escalada E, Cobo J, et al. Can treatment with statins have a negative influence on the tolerance of mandibular advancement devices? Sleep Breath. 2016;20(4):1363–6. https://doi.org/10.1007/s11325-016-1399-8.
61. Marklund M. Long-term efficacy of an oral appliance in early treated patients with obstructive sleep apnea. Sleep Breath. 2016;20(2):689–94. https://doi.org/10.1007/s11325-015-1280-1.
62. Pantin CC, Hillman DR, Tennant M. Dental side effects of an oral device to treat snoring and obstructive sleep apnea. Sleep. 1999;22(2):237–40. https://doi.org/10.1093/sleep/22.2.237.
63. El-Solh AA, Moitheennazima B, Akinnusi ME, Churder PM, Lafornara AM. Combined oral appliance and positive airway pressure therapy for obstructive sleep apnea: a pilot study. Sleep Breath. 2011;15:203–8. https://doi.org/10.1007/s11325-010-0437-1.
64. Dieltjens M, Vroegop AV, Verbruggen AE, et al. A promising concept of combination therapy for positional obstructive sleep apnea. Sleep Breath. 2014;19(2):637–44. https://doi.org/10.1007/s11325-014-1068-8.

Surgical Evaluation and Airway Assessment of Patients with OSA

3

Anastasiya Quimby and Salam O. Salman

3.1 Introduction

Obstructive sleep apnea is the most common sleep-related breathing disorder in the world, with its prevalence continuing to increase. Sleep-disordered breathing is a continuum beginning with primary snoring to upper airway resistance syndrome to obstructive sleep apnea and ending with obesity-hypoventilation syndrome. Obstructive sleep apnea is further subdivided into mild, moderate, and severe. Although the pathophysiology of obstructive sleep apnea is multifactorial, it is generally due to obstruction or collapse of the upper airway at one or more of the following levels: the nasopharynx, oropharynx, and hypopharynx [1]. Some sleep physicians also include the larynx as the fourth anatomical location for possible site of obstruction in patients with OSA [2]. In order to accurately evaluate patients with OSA, one must have an understanding of the relevant surgical anatomy.

3.2 Relevant Surgical Anatomy

From the nares, air funnels through two valves, which are the narrowest point of passage. Deformities and the collapse of the alar cartilage can obstruct or stenose the external nasal valves. Internal nasal valve collapse or constriction can also lead to decreased nasopharyngeal airflow, which can easily be evaluated clinically by performing a Cottle test. Between the external and internal nasal valves, septal deviations and enlarged inferior turbinates can further contribute to obstruction of flow. Maxillary constriction, a high-arched palate, and dental occlusal crossbites will further narrow the nasal floor and constrict air flow. The oropharynx is the most

A. Quimby · S. O. Salman (✉)
Department of Oral and Maxillofacial Surgery, College of Medicine, University of Florida—Jacksonville, Jacksonville, FL, USA
e-mail: salam.salman@jax.ufl.edu; anastasiya.quimby@jax.ufl.edu

S. O. Salman (ed.), *Modern Management of Obstructive Sleep Apnea*, https://doi.org/10.1007/978-3-030-11443-5_3

common site of obstruction in patients with OSA [3]. This area extends from the soft palate to the epiglottis and includes the palatine tonsils, posterior tongue, and pharyngeal constrictors and is influenced by the position of the maxilla and mandible, soft palate, and adenotonsillar region. A retrognathic maxilla and/or mandible can lead to decreased space posterior to the hard palate and tongue. The thickness and length of the soft palate, lymphoid hyperplasia especially in the adolescent patient, and certain craniofacial skeletal abnormalities all contribute to airway flow deficiencies. Airway flow can be unintentionally inhibited postsurgically, such as status-post cleft palate repair surgeries or pharyngeal flaps. Chronic OSA has even been shown to cause the palate to thicken, elongate, and descend, further worsening airway flow. The hypopharyngeal region extends from the cephalad border of the epiglottis to the cricoid cartilage inferiorly. Lingual tonsillar hypertrophy and a lax epiglottis can lead to decreased airway space and obstruction in this region. Constriction in these areas is not only limited to anterior-posterior dimensions but lateral and concentric dimensions, all of which can contribute to upper airway obstruction.

3.3 Clinical Assessment

The assessment of patients with suspected sleep-disordered breathing should begin with examining the patient's history, comorbidities, and basic sleep questionnaires, preferably with their partner present. A comprehensive sleep history should include an evaluation for snoring, witness apneas, excessive or early daytime somnolence, total sleep time, and assessment of sleepiness severity by the Epworth Sleepiness Scale (ESS) [4]. An ESS of ten or greater warrants further investigation as it indicates an increased likelihood of sleep-disordered breathing. Another simple questionnaire that can easily be completed, which includes some physical findings as well, is the STOP-Bang Questionnaire [5]. This questionnaire consists of four questions (STOP), snoring, tiredness, observed apneas, and treatment for high blood pressure, and four clinical findings (Bang), BMI > 35, age > 50, neck circumference greater than 40 cm or 16 in., and male gender. The probability of moderate to severe OSA increases in direct proportion to an increased STOP-Bang score. When categorizing moderate to severe OSA, those with scores less than 3 can be considered low risk, and those with scores 5 or greater as high risk [6]. Along with these questionnaires and review of sleep history, clinical findings associated with OSA should be examined. Common clinical exam findings in patients with OSA include but are not limited to the following: nasal abnormalities, mandibular micro- or retrognathia, high-arched palate, tonsillar hypertrophy, elongated soft palate, macroglossia, obtuse thyromental angle, large neck circumference, and obesity.

Beginning with the nasal exam, assessment for the following clinical findings should be performed:

- External and internal nasal valve collapse
- Septal deviation
- Turbinate and/or mucosal hypertrophy

Oropharyngeal, maxillary, and mandibular skeletal exam signs consistent with an increased risk of having OSA are as follows:

- Constricted maxilla
- High-arched palate
- Elongated soft palate/uvula
- Narrowing of tonsillar pillars
- Adenotonsillar hypertrophy (grade 3 or 4) (Fig. 3.1)
- Micro- and retrognathia
- Microgenia

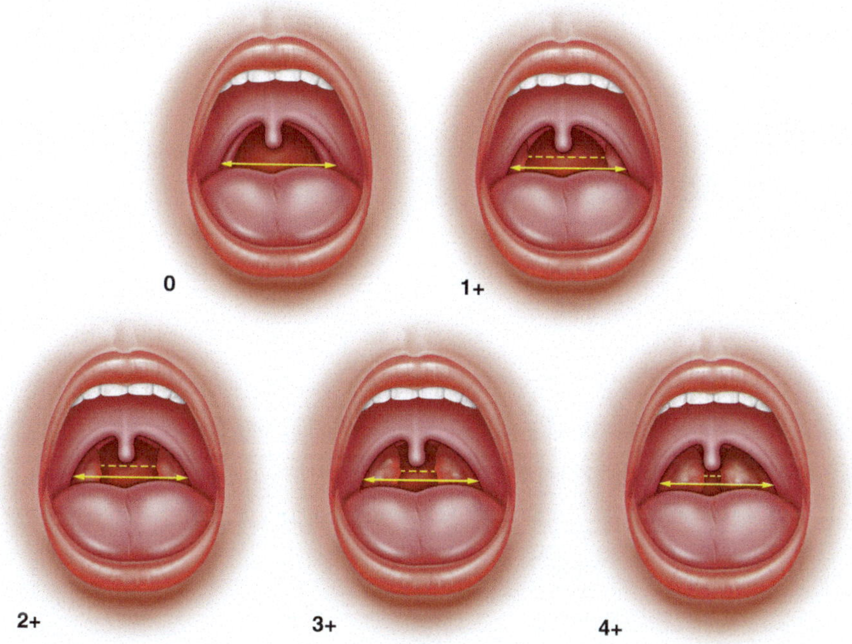

Tonsil size is most often described on a scale from 0 to 5:

- 0 – Tonsils are entirely within the tonsillar pillar, or previously removed by surgery.
- 1+ – Tonsils occupy less than 25 percent of the lateral dimension of the oropharynx, as measured between the anterior tonsillar pillars (solid yellow arrow).
- 2+ – Tonsils occupy 26 to 50 percent of the lateral dimension of the oropharynx.
- 3+ – Tonsils occupy 51 to 75 percent of the lateral dimension of the oropharynx.
- 4+ – Tonsils occupy more than 75 percent of the lateral dimension of the oropharynx.

Fig. 3.1 Brodsky Tonsil Grading Scale

- Modified Mallampati III or IV (inability to visualize posterior oropharyngeal wall) (Fig. 3.2)
- Friedman tongue position III or IV (Fig. 3.3)

Hypopharyngeal exam findings are difficult to assess clinically without the aid of fiber-optic endoscopy, but an enlarged neck circumference, short neck, and low hyoid positions should be clues to the practitioner of the patient's

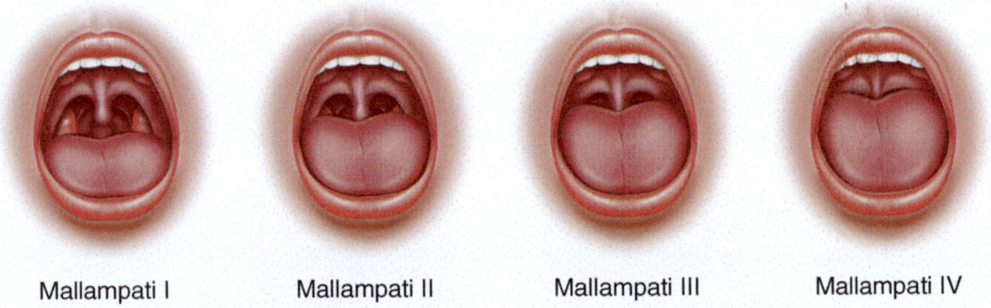

Fig. 3.2 Modified Mallampati Scale

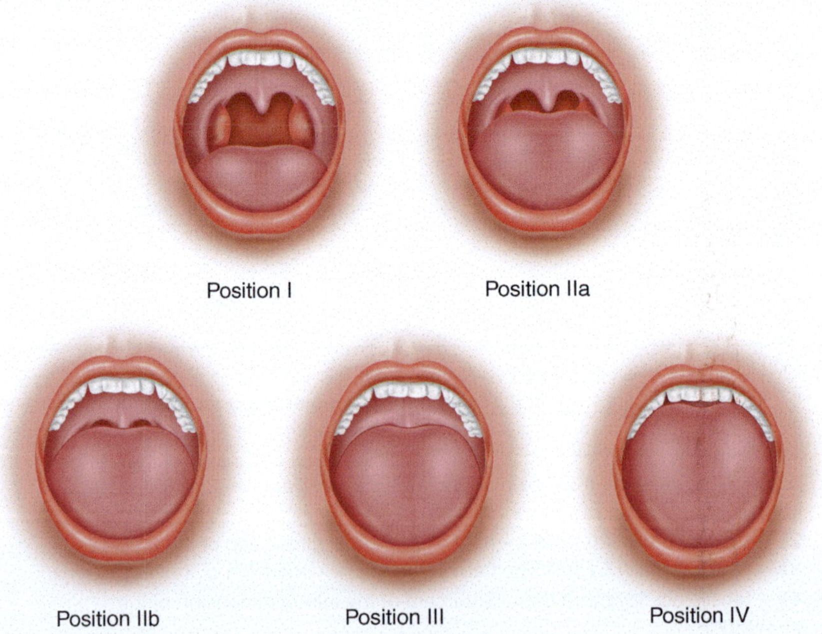

Fig. 3.3 Friedman Tongue Position

Stages	Friedman Tongue Position	Tonsil Size	BMI
I	I, IIa, IIb	3 or 4	<40
II	I, IIa, IIb III or IV	0, 1, or 2 3 or 4	<40 <40
III	III or IV	0, 1, or 2	<40
IV	All	All	>40

Fig. 3.4 Friedman Staging System

higher risk for having upper airway obstruction. Masses or lesions at any location in the upper airway can also lead to obstruction and require further evaluation.

Prior to proceeding with further investigations, such as endoscopy and radiographic imaging, based on clinical exam findings, the Friedman Staging System (FSS) can be utilized to guide surgical interventions and accurately predict the success of surgical outcomes (Fig. 3.4). FSS combines Friedman tongue position (I–IV), tonsil size (0–4), and BMI and separates them into four stages [7]. This system was originally devised to predict surgical success of uvulopalatopharyngoplasty (UPPP) but is a useful assessment and documentation tool for any patient undergoing surgical intervention for the treatment of OSA.

3.4 Upper Airway Endoscopy

Along with a comprehensive history and physical exam, it is imperative to perform flexible nasopharyngoscopy to completely assess the upper airway in detail. This can be performed both awake and asleep, i.e., drug-induced. There are benefits and limitations to both approaches.

Drug-induced sleep endoscopy (DICE) involves the assessment of the upper airway during pharmacologically induced sleep with agents such as propofol, midazolam, dexmedetomidine, and/or opioids. Kezirian et al. introduced a new classification system for obstruction during DICE in 2011 [8]. The VOTE classification not only localizes the site of obstruction but also defines it in regard to degree of obstruction and configuration (i.e., anterior-posterior (AP), lateral, and/or concentric). The agents used to induce sleep intrinsically lead to decreased tone of pharyngeal airway musculature and impart the risk of inducing complete airway obstruction requiring airway protective interventions. Another limitation to DICE is the inability to have the patient perform a Mueller's maneuver to assess for site(s) of obstruction. In 2017, a European position paper on DICE was updated with general recommendations on performing and evaluating sleep endoscopy of OSA [9]. DICE should be performed in an operating room or endoscopy suite setting, after the patient has undergone a type 1, 2, or 3 sleep study. The European position paper also recommends the use of propofol and midazolam together or midazolam alone as the sedative agent. Positioning should mimic the patient's natural sleep position as well. Regarding classification systems, no consensus was obtained; however, the

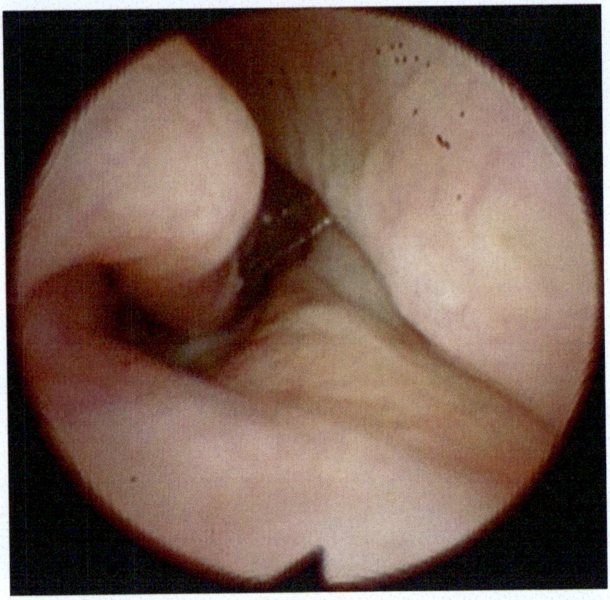

Fig. 3.5 Intranasal image from nasopharyngeal endoscopy

VOTE classification system was recommended along with including a grading system for degree of obstruction/collapse [9].

Awake endoscopy is performed while the patient is supine. The patient's position can then be changed to perform Mueller's maneuver. Mueller's maneuver is performed while the patient is upright with a closed mouth and pinched nose with maximum inspiration. The increased intraluminal negative pressure with this maneuver attempts to duplicate the sleep-related pressure changes to more accurately assess the presence of dynamic upper airway collapse. The limitation of awake endoscopy is the inability to visualize the anatomical site(s) of obstruction during sleep, pharmacologically induced or not.

Both techniques, however, allow for visualization of the entire upper airway in detail as well as aid in objectively assessing surgical changes and/or success in treating the site(s) of obstruction postoperatively [10]. Endoscopic examination allows the practitioner to visualize the nasal cavity, assessing for septal deviation, turbinate hypertrophy, nasal polyps, etc. (Fig. 3.5) [11]. Working further into the nasopharynx, assessment of velopharyngeal obstruction can be performed. Collapse in all three dimensions, AP, lateral, and concentric, can occur at this site (Fig. 3.6). Entering the oropharynx, the lateral pharyngeal walls and tonsillar pillars can be assessed for lateral collapse and/or adenotonsillar hypertrophy. And finally, the base of the tongue can be evaluated for both AP collapse and lingual tonsillar hypertrophy (LTH), along with assessment of the epiglottis for laxity leading to airway obstruction (Fig. 3.7). Lingual tonsillar hypertrophy can be graded on a scale from 0 to 4 as follows (Fig. 3.8) [7]:

- Grade 0—complete absence of lymphoid tissue
- Grade 1—lymphoid tissue scattered over the tongue base

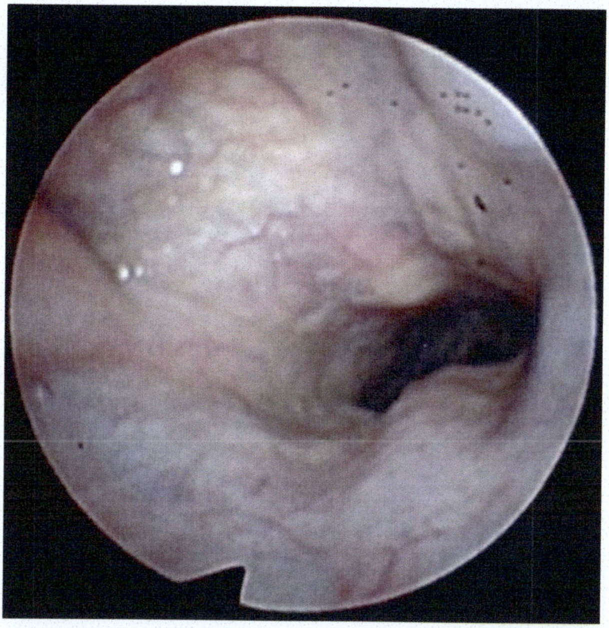

Fig. 3.6 Soft palate image from nasopharyngeal endoscopy

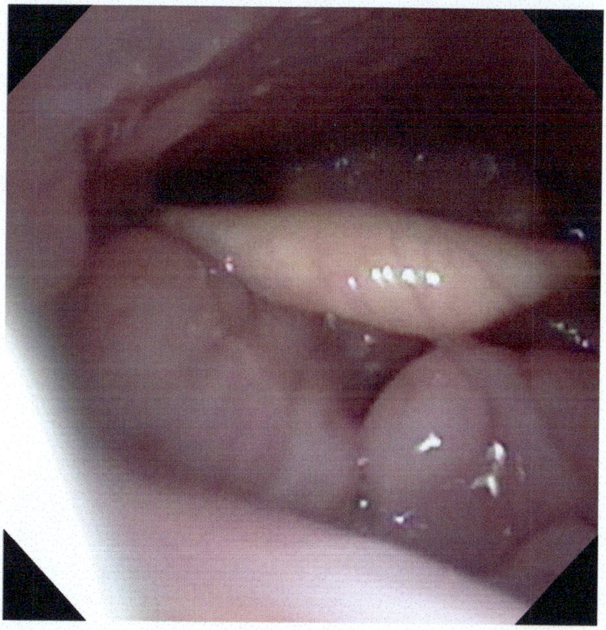

Fig. 3.7 Lingual tonsil image from nasopharyngeal endoscopy

- Grade 2—lymphoid tissue covering the entirety of the tongue base with limited vertical thickness
- Grade 3—significantly raised lymphoid tissue (5–10 mm thick)
- Grade 4—lymphoid tissue 1 cm or more thick rising over the epiglottis

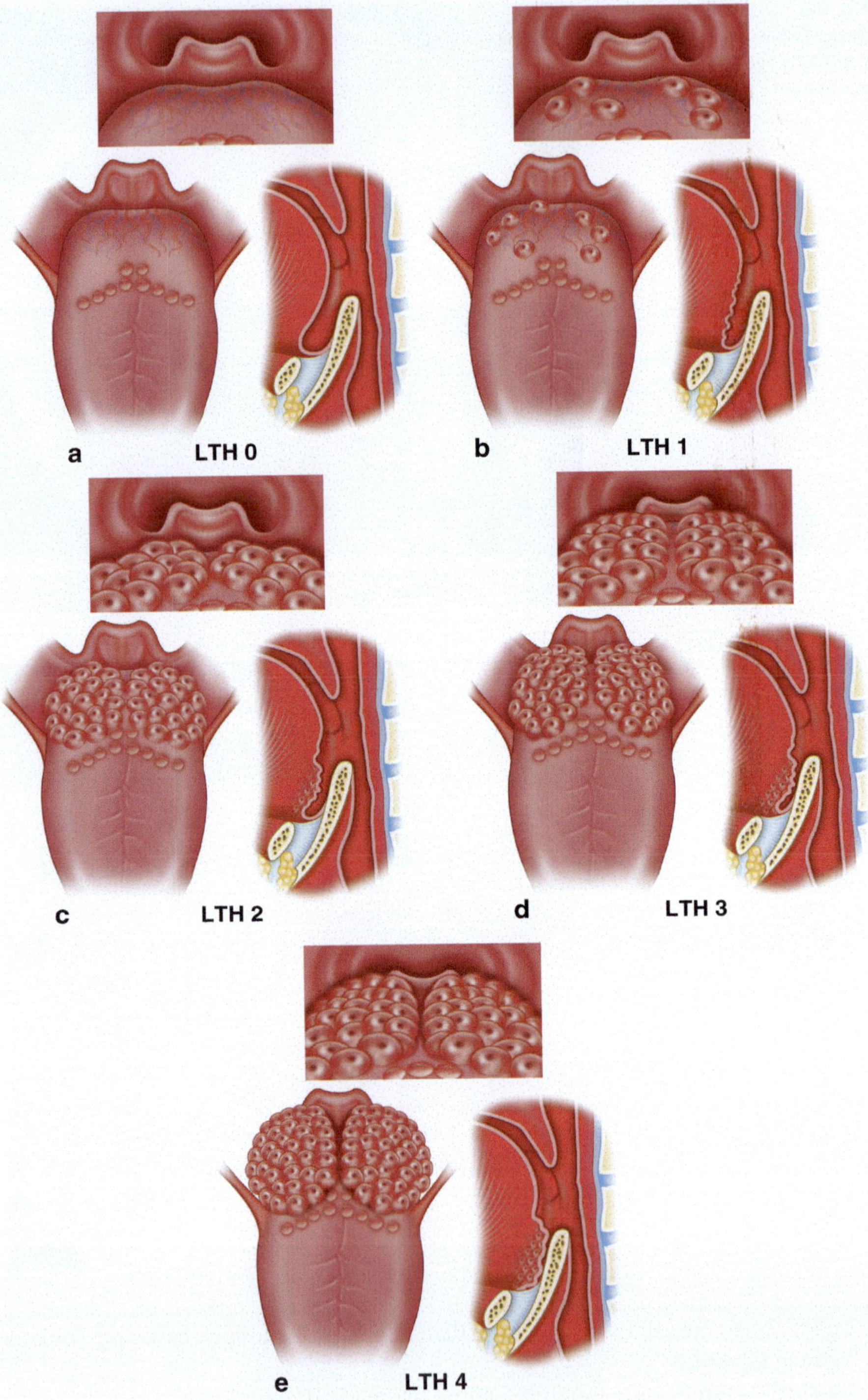

Fig. 3.8 Lingual Tonsil Hypertrophy (LTH) Grading Scale

A meta-analysis performed by Lee and Cho in 2018 concluded that upon endoscopic examination, patients with OSA were more likely to have multilevel obstruction rather than single-site obstruction [12]. Of the patients included in the meta-analysis, 84.1% had obstruction at the soft palate, 51.6% at the base of the tongue, 34.3% at the epiglottis, and 32.8% at the tonsils [12]. This further demonstrates the importance of performing nasopharyngeal endoscopy for evaluation of patients with OSA, due to the multilevel location of upper airway collapsibility and inability to appropriately assess these anatomical sites with only a clinical exam.

3.5 Radiographic Imaging

There are several options for radiographic imaging of patients with OSA. Depending on the sleep physician's preference and accessibility to certain types of imaging, multiple modalities can be utilized. The quickest and cheapest option for imaging is a lateral cephalogram (Fig. 3.9). This option is easily accessible to most oral and maxillofacial surgeons and is a quick tool to assess the anterior-posterior dimension of the patient's upper airway. Mandibular or maxillary position can easily be assessed with this form of imaging, and patients with skeletal deficiencies are more prone to have airway obstruction retropalatally and at the base of the tongue [13]. Several measurements can be obtained from a lateral cephalogram that can indicate the likelihood or increased risk of a patient having OSA, including, but not limited to, PNS-P (posterior nasal spine to caudal aspect of palate) length greater than 37 ± 3 mm, MP-H (mandibular plane to hyoid) greater than 15.4 ± 3 mm, and PAS (posterior airway space as measured from the continuation of a line B-point to Gonion to the posterior pharyngeal wall) less than 11 ± 1 mm. Although this modality is an upright, static, two-dimensional image, Riley and colleagues demonstrated a statistically significant correlation between PAS measured on lateral cephalograms and pharyngeal airway volume measured on computer tomography scans [14].

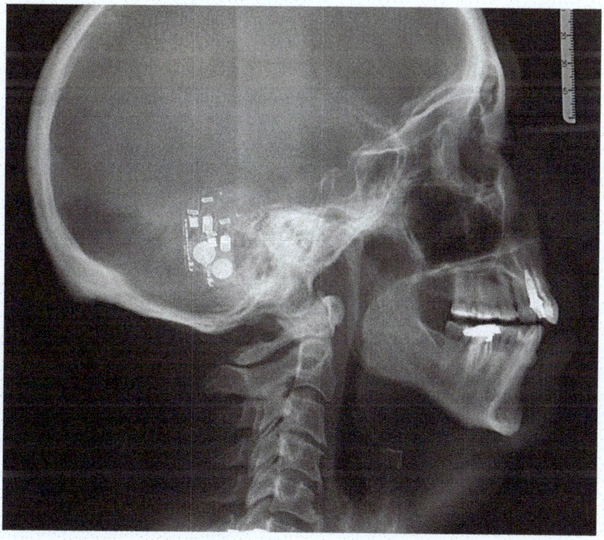

Fig. 3.9 Lateral cephalogram demonstrating decreased airway space and low-positioned hyoid

Another radiographic option, also commonly accessible to many practitioners, is computed tomography. An upright cone beam computed tomography (CBCT) provides more information than a two-dimensional lateral cephalogram. Visualization of the upper airway three-dimensionally can provide the specific location of airway obstruction in both anterior-posterior and lateral dimensions (Fig. 3.10) [15]. Airway space measurements, including volume and cross-sectional area, have been shown to be quite accurate by use of CBCT scans. Although this is a static image, and predominately completed in an upright position, multivariate analysis shows airway narrowing on CBCT to be predictive of an elevated degree of obstruction [16]. CBCT imaging is also beneficial and utilized for virtual surgical planning in cases requiring skeletal surgery, i.e., maxillomandibular and/or genioglossal advancement. Postsurgical images can be used to compare and quantify an increase in upper airway space, which can then be correlated to the patient's decrease in AHI.

Conventional computed tomography (CT) in supine position, although more time-consuming and costly, can also be utilized for preoperative assessment of the patient undergoing upper airway obstruction surgery (Fig. 3.11). In regard to base of the tongue procedures, the location of the dorsal lingual artery can be visualized and incorporated in the surgical plan to decrease the risk of injury. Three-dimensional measurements similar to CBCT images can be obtained as well, with visualization of anterior-posterior and lateral collapse. Li et al. demonstrated a relationship between upper airway area and probability of suffering from OSA based on CT analysis. They concluded that there is a high probability of severe OSA with an airway area of less than 52 mm^2, an intermediate probability if the airway is between 52 and 110 mm^2, and a low probability if the airway is greater than 110 mm^2 [17].

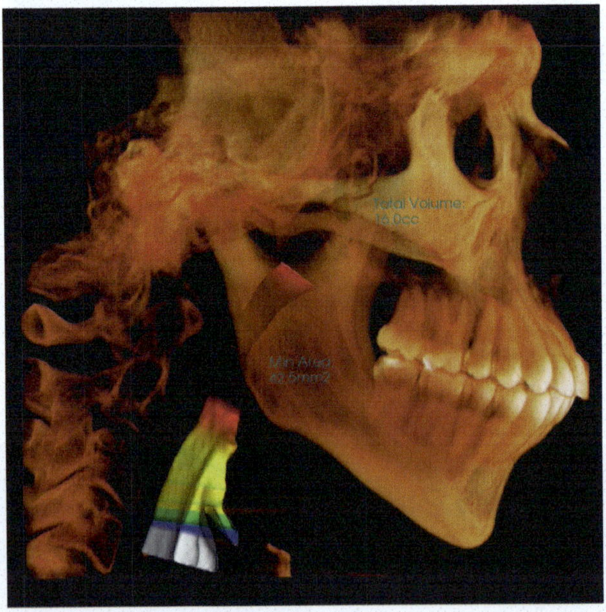

Fig. 3.10 Cone beam CT scan 3D airway assessment [Software—Invivo6, Anatomage, San Jose, CA]

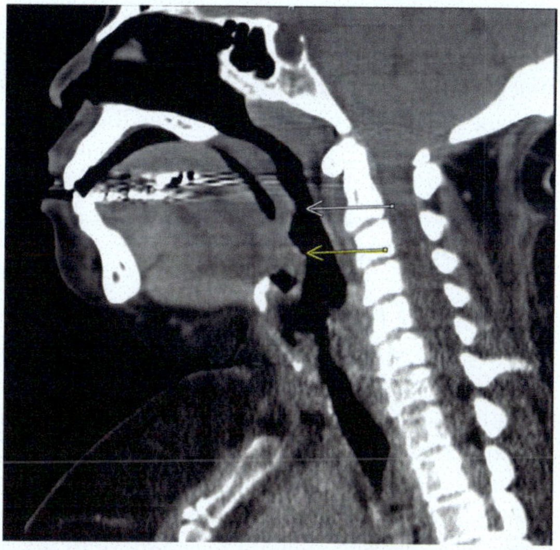

Fig. 3.11 CT scan indicating lingual tonsillar hypertrophy and elongated soft palate

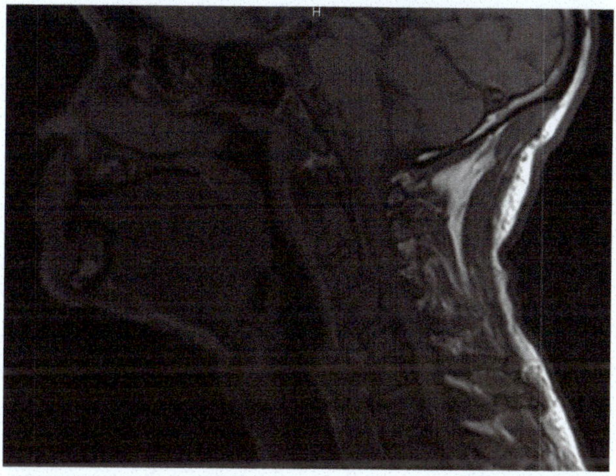

Fig. 3.12 MRI demonstrating and elongated soft palate and retropalatal obstruction

A common critic of radiographic imaging is that they do not accurately capture airway anatomy during obstruction or airway collapse. Recent studies have been performed with drug-induced CT imaging, similar to the concept of DICE [18]. Results demonstrate the vast majority of patients (89%) exhibit multilevel obstruction, with the most common sites of obstruction occurring in the retropalatal level (86%), retroglossal level (57%), oropharyngeal lateral walls (49%), and epiglottis (26%) [19].

Finally, magnetic resonance imaging (MRI) can be utilized for further evaluation of the upper airway (Fig. 3.12) [20]. This modality is by far the most time-consuming and costly option but can provide precise analysis of the upper airway during obstruction. Kavcic et al. published a study utilizing this modality during natural sleep as monitored by electroencephalogram in an attempt to dynamically capture the specific site(s) of obstruction. Their group found that in 47% of patients, the palate was attached to the tongue base and both moved posteriorly to obstruct the airway, in 33% the soft palate was detached from the tongue base and solely moved posteriorly, and in 20% of the patients, both mechanisms of obstruction were noted [21].

3.6 Summary

A thorough and detailed upper airway examination is critical for patients undergoing surgical management of sleep-disordered breathing. The pathophysiology of obstructive sleep apnea is multifactorial and is most commonly due to obstruction or collapse of the upper airway at multiple levels. A complete surgical evaluation includes a comprehensive physical exam, nasopharyngeal endoscopy, and radiographic imaging. Unfortunately, beyond tracheostomy, there is not a single treatment that predictably leads to a cure for all patients; therefore treating patients with a "one-size-fits-all" mentality is contrary to the standard of care. Treatment should be individually targeted for patients based on their OSA severity and clinical, endoscopic, and radiographic findings to target and address the specific site(s) of obstruction.

References

1. Chebbo A, Tfaili A, Ghamande S. Anatomy and physiology of obstructive sleep apnea. Sleep Med Clin. 2013;8:425.
2. Vicini C, De Vito A, Benazzo M, Frassineti S, Campanini A, Frasconi P, Mira E. The nose oropharynx hypopharynx and larynx (NOHL) classification: a new system of diagnostic standardized examination for OSAHS patients. Eur Arch Otorhinolaryngol. 2012;269:1297.
3. Schwab RJ, Gefter WB, Hoffman EA, Gupta KB, Pack AI. Dynamic upper airway imaging during awake respiration in normal subjects and patients with sleep disordered breathing. Am Rev Respir Dis. 1993;148:1385.
4. Johns MW. A new method for measuring daytime sleepiness: the Epworth sleepiness scale. Sleep. 1991;14:540.
5. Chung F, Yegneswaran B, Liao P, Chung SA, Vairavanathan S, Islam S, Khajehdehi A, Shapiro CM. STOP questionnaire: a tool to screen patients for obstructive sleep apnea. Anesthesiology. 2008;108:812.
6. Chung F, Abdullah HR, Liao P. STOP-bang questionnaire: a practical approach to screen for obstructive sleep Apnea. Chest. 2016;149:631.
7. Friedman M, Salapatas AM, Bonzelaar LB. Updated Friedman staging system for obstructive sleep apnea. Adv Otorhinolaryngol. 2017;80:41.
8. Kezirian EJ, Hohenhorst W, de Vries N. Drug-induced sleep endoscopy: the VOTE classification. Eur Arch Otorhinolaryngol. 2011;268:1233.
9. De Vito A, Carrasco Llatas M, Ravesloot MJ, Kotecha B, De Vries N, Hamans E, Maurer J, Bosi M, Blumen M, Heiser C, Herzog M, Montevecchi F, Corso RM, Braghiroli A, Gobbi R, Vroegop A, Vonk PE, Hohenhorst W, Piccin O, Sorrenti G, Vanderveken OM, Vicini C. European position paper on drug-induced sleep endoscopy: 2017 update. Clin Otolaryngol. 2018;43:1541.

10. Wang Y, Sun C, Cui X, Guo Y, Wang Q, Liang H. The role of drug-induced sleep endoscopy: predicting and guiding upper airway surgery for adult OSA patients. Sleep Breath. 2018;22:925.
11. Sethukumar P, Kotecha B. Tailoring surgical interventions to treat obstructive sleep apnoea: one size does not fit all. Breathe (Sheff). 2018;14:e84.
12. Lee EJ, Cho JH. Meta-analysis of obstruction site observed with drug-induced sleep endoscopy in patients with obstructive sleep apnea. Laryngoscope. 2019. https://doi.org/10.1002/lary.27320. https://onlinelibrary.wiley.com/action/showCitFormats?doi=10.1002%2Flary.27320.
13. Riley R, Guilleminault C, Herran J, Powell N. Cephalometric analyses and flow-volume loops in obstructive sleep apnea patients. Sleep. 1983;6:303.
14. Riley R, Guilleminault C, Powell N, Simmons FB. Palatopharyngoplasty failure, cephalometric roentgenograms, and obstructive sleep apnea. Otolaryngol Head Neck Surg. 1985;93:240.
15. Camacho M, Capasso R, Schendel S. Airway changes in obstructive sleep apnoea patients associated with a supine versus an upright position examined using cone beam computed tomography. J Laryngol Otol. 2014;128:824.
16. Yamashina A, Tanimoto K, Sutthiprapaporn P, Hayakawa Y. The reliability of computed tomography (CT) values and dimensional measurements of the oropharyngeal region using cone beam CT: comparison with multidetector CT. Dentomaxillofac Radiol. 2008;37:245.
17. Li H-Y, Chen N-H, Wang C-R, Shu Y-H, Wang P-C. Use of 3-dimensional computed tomography scan to evaluate upper airway patency for patients undergoing sleep-disordered breathing surgery. Otolaryngol Head Neck Surg. 2003;129:336.
18. Lee LA, Wang CJ, Lo YL, Huang CG, Kuo IC, Lin WN, Hsin LJ, Fang TJ, Li HY. Drug-induced sleep computed tomography-directed upper airway surgery for obstructive sleep apnea: a pilot study. Otolaryngol Head Neck Surg. 2018:194599818800288.
19. Li H-Y, Lo Y-L, Wang C-J, Hsin L-J, Lin W-N, Fang T-J, Lee L-A. Dynamic drug-induced sleep computed tomography in adults with obstructive sleep apnea. Sci Rep. 2016;6:35849.
20. Ciscar MA, Juan G, Martinez V, Ramon M, Lloret T, Minguez J, Armengot M, Marin J, Basterra J. Magnetic resonance imaging of the pharynx in OSA patients and healthy subjects. Eur Respir J. 2001;17:79.
21. Kavcic P, Koren A, Koritnik B, Fajdiga I, Groselj LD. Sleep magnetic resonance imaging with electroencephalogram in obstructive sleep apnea syndrome. Laryngoscope. 2015;125:1485.

Nasal Surgery

4

Anthony M. Bunnell and Tirbod Fattahi

4.1 Introduction

Obstructive sleep apnea (OSA) is recognized as a spectrum of signs and symptoms arising from obstruction of airflow somewhere in the nasopharyngeal, oropharyngeal, and/or hypopharyngeal regions. This disease has been thoroughly delineated in other chapters in this textbook. Furthermore, in another chapter, nasal endoscopy was described as an important diagnostic modality in the evaluation of patients with OSA. One of the common sites of airflow obstruction in patients with OSA is the nasal complex. Nasal airflow obstruction can also be seen in many subsets of the population without any evidence of OSA, so diagnosing nasal airflow issues in patients with OSA should not be a surprise. The most common sites of airflow obstruction within the nasal complex include external and internal nasal valve areas, nasal tip, nasal septum, and nasal turbinates. Mucosal hypertrophy, as a result of environmental insults such as pollen, pollution, and seasonal allergies can also contribute to this airflow deficit. The purpose of this chapter is to discuss the surgical management of airflow obstruction within the nasal cavity in patients suffering from OSA.

A. M. Bunnell
Division of Head and Neck Surgery, Department of Oral and Maxillofacial Surgery, College of Medicine, University of Florida—Jacksonville, Jacksonville, FL, USA
e-mail: Anthony.Bunnell@Jax.Ufl.Edu

T. Fattahi (✉)
Department of Oral and Maxillofacial Surgery, College of Medicine, University of Florida—Jacksonville, Jacksonville, FL, USA
e-mail: Tirbod.Fattahi@Jax.Ufl.Edu

S. O. Salman (ed.), *Modern Management of Obstructive Sleep Apnea*,
https://doi.org/10.1007/978-3-030-11443-5_4

4.2 Preoperative Evaluation

The essence of the evaluation of the patient with a nasal complaint with OSA is no different than any other cosmetic or functional procedure. While patients' wishes are certainly an important factor, correlation of patients' concerns with the clinicians' observations and diagnoses are imperative. It is also important to recognize that nasal obstruction may coexist with other anatomical sites of airflow obstruction outside of the nasal cavity [1–3].

Standardized photographs are necessary for all rhinoplasty patients regardless of cosmetic or functional complaints. Frontal, three-quarters, profile, and submental views are the absolute minimum required photos. During the evaluation process, specific history of previous nasal trauma, nasal or septal surgery, and/or sinus surgery must be ascertained. Nasal endoscopy (discussed in a previous chapter) is indicated in all patients with OSA, and computed tomography might be of benefit in patients with previous sinus or nasal surgery or previous trauma (Fig. 4.1).

Once the history has been obtained, the physical examination begins. An overall assessment of the entire nasal complex must be taken into consideration; is it deviated, is it wide, and does the nose look too big or too small (over-rotated, under-projected, etc.)? Oftentimes, nasal complex deviation is indicative of septal deviations. Asymmetrical nostrils are also telltale signs of caudal septal deviation. Any underlying cartilaginous or bony irregularities should also be noted. Evaluation of the specific areas of the nasal airflow obstruction is then performed. These areas include the external nasal valve area, nasal tip, the internal naval valve areas, nasal septum, and inferior turbinates. Pathology and/or irregularities along any of these sites can certainly interfere with the normal pathway of airflow. Another important aspect of the physical exam is the evaluation of the soft tissue envelope of the nose. Thick, oily, and sebaceous overlying skin can impact the underlying cartilaginous support areas. This is analogous to a heavy person laying in a hammock; due to the additional weight, the hammock will tend to hang much lower.

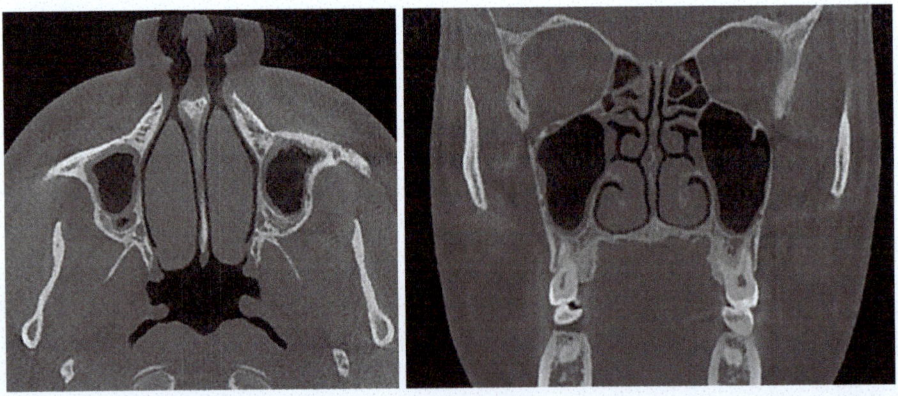

Fig. 4.1 CT scan demonstrating enlarged inferior turbinates

Evaluation of the external nasal valves begins by observing normal breathing through the nostrils. The main structural support of the external valve area are the paired lateral and medial crura. Many patients with weakness of the lower lateral cartilages, or weakness of the alar rim perimeter, will display an inward indentation of the lower lateral cartilages upon normal breathing (Fig. 4.2). Some patients will complain that their breathing improves if they "hold their nasal tip upward" (Fig. 4.3). Further assessment of the external valves can also be done by testing the integrity of the lower cartilages by placing a cotton tip applicator under the cartilage and determining how rigid or stiff the cartilages are. Next the integrity of the internal nasal valve is assessed via a Cottle's test. The internal nasal valve, the narrowest portion of the nasal passages, is comprised of the attachment of the upper lateral cartilages to the dorsal septum. This attachment creates two valves, one on each side, with a patency angle of approximately 15° (Fig. 4.4). Since the valves are so small, any irregularity in this area can lead to restriction of airflow. The Cottle's test is performed by occluding one nostril and having the patient breathe in and out of the other nostril. Cheek tissue on the ipsilateral side (breathing side) is then pulled laterally while breathing; if breathing significantly improves, the test is positive, and there is collapse of the internal nasal valve on that side. This collapse or narrowing can be unilateral or bilateral. Endoscopic and speculum examination of the internal

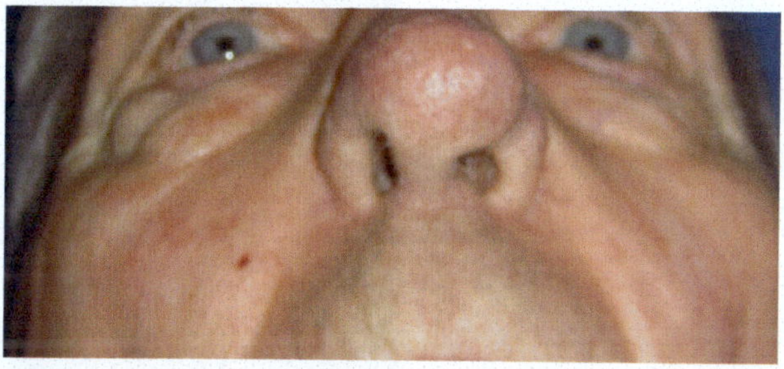

Fig. 4.2 Collapse of right nares upon deep inspiration

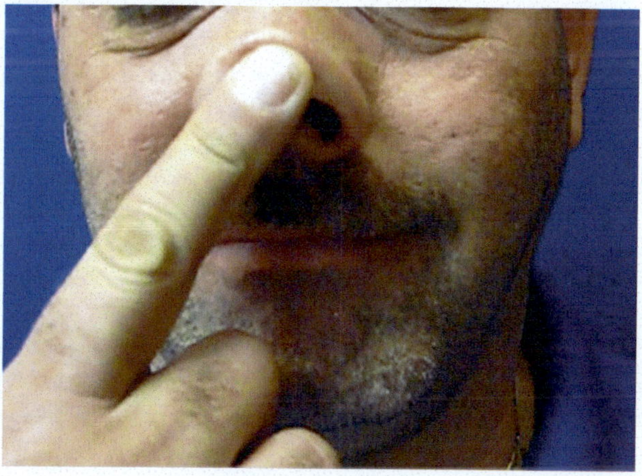

Fig. 4.3 Evidence of lack of nasal tip support; patient holds his nasal tip up in order to breath

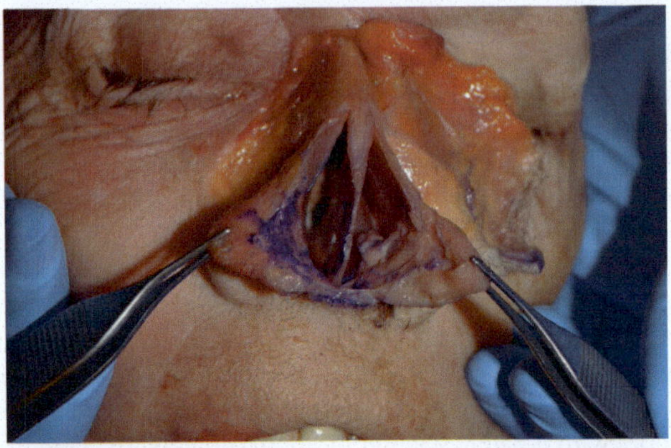

Fig. 4.4 Cadaveric specimen demonstrating bilateral internal nasal valves

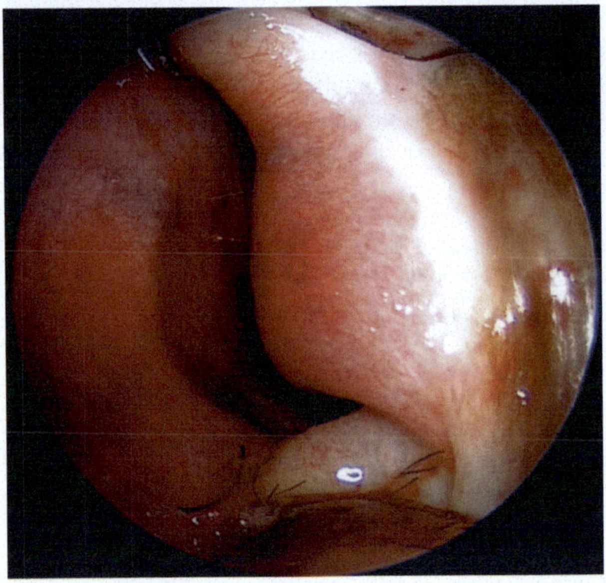

Fig. 4.5 Endoscopic view of enlarged left inferior turbinate

nose is done next. Septal deviation, turbinate hypertrophy, presence of conchal bullosa (air pockets within turbinate bones), and an evaluation of the patency of the nasal airway all the way into the nasopharynx are assessed (Fig. 4.5). At the completion of the physical exam, a complete list of diagnoses is formulated.

4.3 Surgical Technique

It is not unusual for patients with nasal obstruction to have multiple sites of airflow restriction. This is no different for a patient with OSA. As previously mentioned, nasal obstruction may coexist with other abnormalities in patients with OSA such as oro- and hypopharyngeal sites of obstruction. Improvement in nasal airflow will undoubtedly improve signs and symptoms associated with OSA.

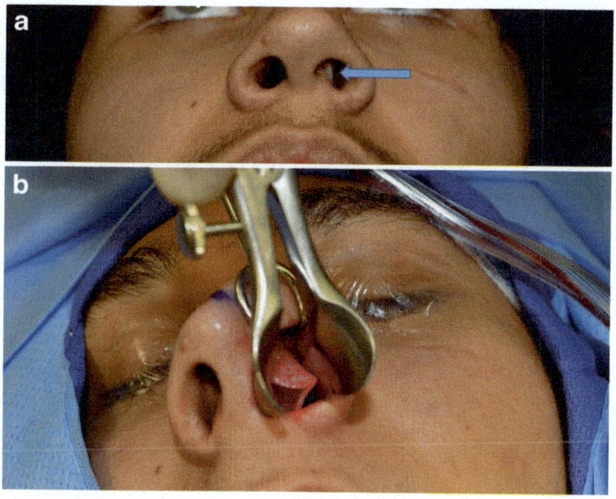

Fig. 4.6 (**a** and **b**) Deviated nasal septum (preoperative—arrow) and intraoperative image. Deviation such as this can cause significant airflow obstruction

Surgical options for nasal surgery in patients for OSA depend on the specific sites of airflow restriction determined in the evaluation process. If the only site of obstruction is the nasal septum, then a simple septoplasty may suffice. Septoplasty can be performed as an isolated procedure or can be combined with a formal functional rhinoplasty (Fig. 4.6). If performed by itself, the surgeon can simply "score" the septum in order to correct deviations within the cartilage or perform a submucous resection of the septum (SMR). SMR involves removal of a portion of the cartilaginous septum in order to eliminate deviation and for grafting purposes during a functional rhinoplasty. When performing a SMR, one must leave a 1 cm "L" strut of remaining cartilage to maintain support of the nasal complex. Isolated septoplasty can significantly improve airflow; it is a predictable procedure with minimal complications if performed correctly [4, 5].

Collapse of the external nasal valve usually requires reinforcement of the lower lateral cartilages and the alar rim. This can be performed via an endonasal or open approach to the nose. Weakness of the lateral crus, a common cause of external collapse, combined with weakness of the alar rim, is addressed with precision placement of structural grafts. These grafts are ideally harvested from the septum during a septoplasty. The author prefers to address external valve issues via an open technique. In doing so, the entire dome is exposed. Attention can be given to specific areas of the nasal tip that may require augmentation. Weakened lower lateral cartilage can be reinforced via placement of batten grafts. These grafts essentially strengthen the overlying cartilage by adding rigidity. Batten grafts can be placed on the dorsal side or underside of the lateral crus. If placed on the dorsal side, care must be taken to ensure that the edges of the graft are not palpable through the overlying soft tissue envelope. Alternatively, a precise pocket can be developed between the nasal mucosa and the lateral crus; the batten graft can then be placed in this pocket (Fig. 4.7). Alar rim weakness can also contribute to an external valve collapse. A weakened rim, especially common in secondary rhinoplasty, can be addressed by placing a narrow cartilage graft (known as rim grafts) within a soft tissue pocket

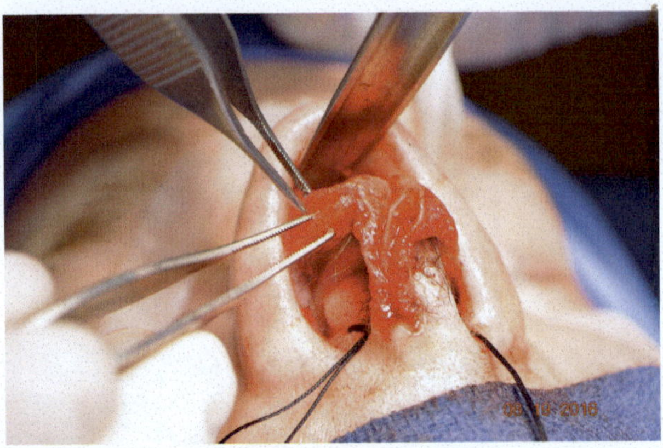

Fig. 4.7 Batten graft placed in between nasal mucosa and right lateral crus

outlining the perimeter of the nares. These maneuvers, especially when coupled with batten grafts, can provide strong structural integrity to the external valve area (Fig. 4.8).

The nasal tip/dome area can also be enhanced by placing a strong columellar strut graft. This graft acts as a "loading bearing wall," decreasing the chance of nasal tip collapse, especially on deep inspiration. This graft is placed precisely between the two medial crura, on top of the anterior nasal spine. It is then sutured to the surrounding cartilages with a mattress suture (Fig. 4.9). A columellar strut graft is mandatory in all open approaches to the nose considering that the open technique violates the transdomal ligament. Transdomal ligaments are a major structural support mechanism on the nasal tip; therefore, reinforcement is required [6].

The internal nasal valve, the confluence of dorsal septum, and upper lateral cartilages can be enhanced by placement of uni- or bilateral spreader grafts. These grafts, originally described by Sheen in 1984 to address mid-vault deficiency, can widen a narrow internal valve. Spreader grafts are procured from a harvested nasal septum and placed between the upper lateral cartilages and the dorsal septum [7, 8]. Again, one must leave a 1 cm "L" strut of remaining cartilage to maintain support of the nasal complex. They are typically 20–30 mm in length and can straighten a nose in addition to providing structural support and improvement in breathing function (Fig. 4.10).

Inferior turbinates can often become quite enlarged, causing a major obstruction to the flow of air within the nasal cavity. This is especially true in patients with septal deviation where the side of the nose away from the deviation will actually undergo a compensatory hypertrophy of the inferior turbinate. Further airflow obstruction can also occur due to creation of "air pockets" known as concha bullosa

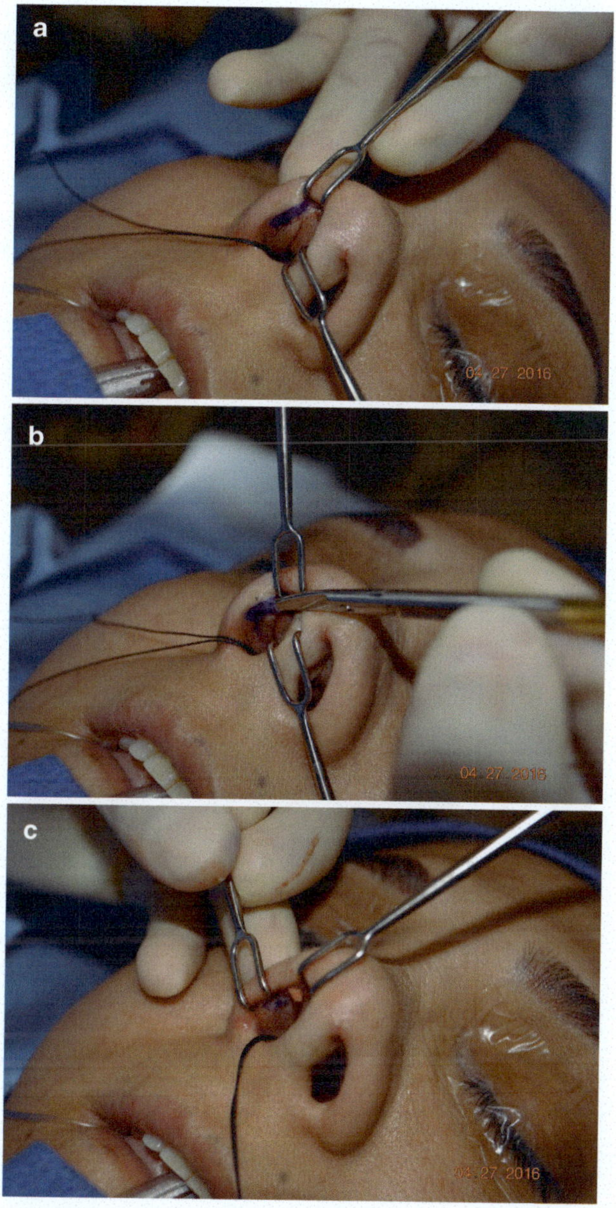

Fig. 4.8 (a–c) Marking, creation, and placement of an alar rim graft

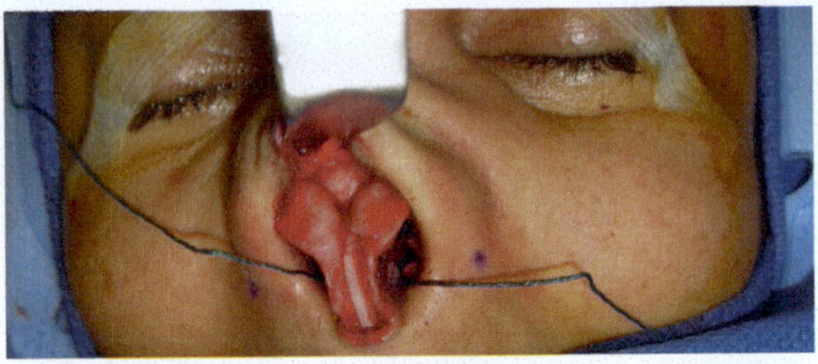

Fig. 4.9 Columellar strut graft in place

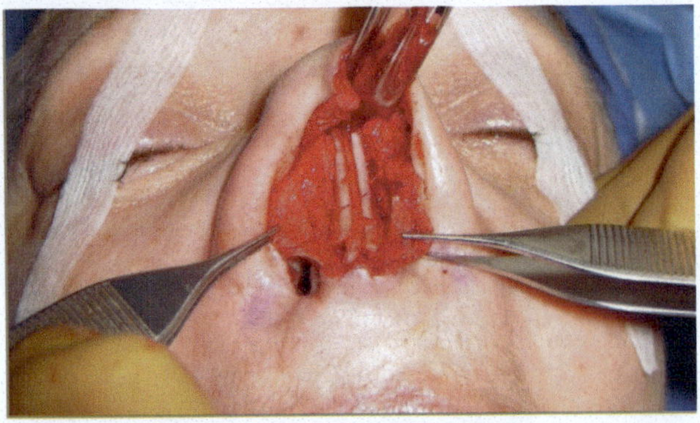

Fig. 4.10 Spreader grafts in place

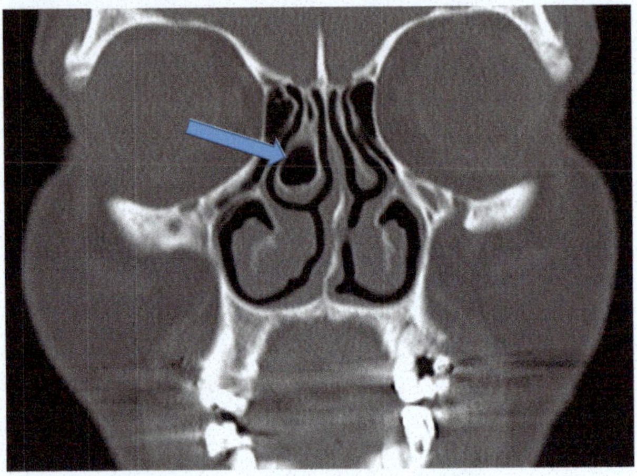

Fig. 4.11 CT scan demonstrating septal deviation, turbinate hypertrophy, and a conchal bullosa (arrow)

(Fig. 4.11). Turbinate hypertrophy and concha bullosa are addressed by "out-fracturing" these areas. Inferior turbinates are a spongy type of bone with lots of trabeculae inside; out-fracturing these bones will diminish their size quite nicely while still maintaining the humidification purposes of the turbinates [9, 10]. Inferior turbinate reduction and/or removal of concha bullosa can be performed as an isolated procedure, combined with a formal rhinoplasty or can be done via a functional endoscopic sinus surgery (FESS).

4.4 Conclusion

As mentioned before, symptoms of OSA can arise from a number of different sites in the head and neck region. Nasal deformities can certainly cause significant airflow obstruction. While patients with OSA may have simultaneous nasal and other site-specific causes of airflow obstruction, addressing the nasal component can significantly decrease the severity of OSA. Nasal surgery in patients with OSA requires a complete nasal evaluation as a component of a comprehensive OSA workup. If performed appropriately, functional nasal surgery can improve nasopharyngeal airflow, decreasing or completely eliminating signs and symptoms of OSA.

References

1. Li HY, Lee LA, Wang PC, Fang TJ, Chen NH. Can nasal surgery improve obstructive sleep apnea: subjective or objective? Am J Rhinol Allergy. 2009;23(6):e51–5.
2. Sufioğlu M, Ozmen OA, Kasapoglu F, Demir UL, Ursavas A, Erişen L, Onart S. The efficacy of nasal surgery in obstructive sleep apnea syndrome: a prospective clinical study. Eur Arch Otorhinolaryngol. 2012;269(2):487–94.
3. Shuaib SW, Undavia S, Lin J, Johnson CM Jr, Stupak HD. Can functional septorhinoplasty independently treat obstructive sleep apnea? Plast Reconstr Surg. 2015;135(6):1554–65.
4. Fattahi T, Quereshy F. Septoplasty: thoughts and considerations. J Oral Maxillofac Surg. 2011;69(12):e528–32.
5. Radulesco T, Penicaud M, Santini L, Thomassin JM, Dessi P, Michel J. Outcomes of septo-rhinoplasty: a new approach comparing functional and aesthetic results. Int J Oral Maxillofac Surg. 2018;47(2):175–9.
6. Fattahi T. Considerations in revision rhinoplasty: lessons learned. Oral Maxillofac Surg Clin North Am. 2011;23(1):101–8.
7. Sheen JH. Spreader graft: a method of reconstructing the roof of the middle nasal vault following rhinoplasty. Plast Reconstr Surg. 1984;73(2):230–9.
8. Fattahi T. Internal nasal valve: significance in nasal air flow. J Oral Maxillofac Surg. 2008;66(9):1921–6.
9. Ishii LE, Tollefson TT, Basura GJ, et al. Clinical practice guideline: improving nasal form and function after rhinoplasty executive summary. Otolaryngol Head Neck Surg. 2017;156(2):205–19. https://doi.org/10.1177/0194599816683156.
10. Valero A, Navarro AM, Del Cuvillo A, et al. Position paper on nasal obstruction: evaluation and treatment. J Investig Allergol Clin Immunol. 2018;28(2):67–90.

Palatal Surgery

5

Stuart Grayson MacKay and Rachelle L. Love

5.1 Introduction

Surgery for adult obstructive sleep apnea (OSA) is part of a changing paradigm in management of what is a complex and morbid condition. Of historic interest, early surgical procedures focused primarily on ablating the palatal structures, intending to create physical space in the upper airway to facilitate breathing. Ikematsu described the first sleep procedure, the uvulopalatoplasty in 1964 [1], but the procedure only garnered popularity amongst surgeons worldwide after Fujita's 1981 publication [2], which detailed his extensive experience using a modification of the original technique. In the same year, Sullivan et al. [3] published a landmark paper introducing continuous positive airway pressure (CPAP) into the treatment of OSA. The role of surgery was then principally as a salvage option for individuals who failed CPAP.

In the subsequent decades, surgical techniques were refined. A variety of procedures, techniques and approaches have been described, each attempting to strike a balance between sufficiently altering the anatomic subsites involved in the individual's disease and avoiding the complications that arise from surgery to the airway, especially in the context of the OSA patient.

Critical to understanding the evolving role of surgery in OSA is an awareness of the interplay of anatomic and non-anatomic factors in the individual patient. Anatomic scoring systems have traditionally been used to predict which patients may improve with surgery, the most widely used of these are the Friedman [4] and Mallampati [5] classifications. However, improved outcomes following surgery are not wholly dependent upon anatomy. The concept of physiologic endo-phenotypes,

S. G. MacKay (✉)
Illawarra Head and Neck Clinic, Wollongong, NSW, Australia
e-mail: alana@illawarraent.com.au

R. L. Love
Department of Otolaryngology, Christchurch Public Hospital, Christchurch, New Zealand
e-mail: Rachelle.Love@cdhb.health.nz

S. O. Salman (ed.), *Modern Management of Obstructive Sleep Apnea*,
https://doi.org/10.1007/978-3-030-11443-5_5

based on the work of Eckert [6] and Malhotra, has challenged traditional descriptions of pathogenesis. Poor outcomes following surgery may occur because predictive tools based solely on anatomy fail to account for the non-anatomical factors in OSA, such as ventilatory control instability and arousal threshold [7]. What is not known is how these physiologic measures can be incorporated into a sound clinical assessment and whether surgery alters underlying physiology.

In the future, the challenge will be to provide individualized treatment, and, in the hands of the sleep surgeon, this means tailoring proven surgical procedures to the individual. There remains a pressing need for effective alternative therapies for OSA beyond CPAP and a need to develop predictive tools to identify those patients who would benefit best from the available surgical treatments.

5.2 Preoperative Evaluation

Patients with sleep-disordered breathing (SDB) should be evaluated by a dedicated sleep physician or surgeon. The evaluation should include taking a comprehensive history, a structured examination and polysomnography. Optimization of device use, such as CPAP or mandibular advancement splint, should be prioritized. Modifying lifestyle factors contributing to SDB including achieving a healthy weight, optimizing sleep hygiene, managing other sleep disorders such as insomnia and addressing associated medical issues are important.

Patients unable to maintain first-line treatment should be considered for surgical intervention. The choice of operation depends on patient, disease and surgeon factors. The challenge in decision-making is trying to apply effective procedures to the individual in the setting of patients who seek surgery as their preferred option.

Patients opting for surgery need to engage in a detailed discussion about the goals, the risks and benefits of surgery and the requirement for ongoing surveillance of their potentially chronic condition even after they have recovered from surgery.

Pre- and postoperative plans for management of the individual patient typically include medical management of blood pressure, analgesia and approaches to limit complications. Theatre and ward staff require specific training in the management of the surgical patient with OSA, including formalization of postoperative orders (albeit ones that are still flexible to the individual patient) and structured plans for a deteriorating patient.

5.3 Surgical Technique

5.3.1 Uvulopalatopharyngoplasty

Uvulopalatopharyngoplasty (UPPP) is the most widely used and researched procedure in OSA surgery [8]. Modifications to the original uvulopalatopharyngoplasty are the result of complications, such as difficulty swallowing, velopharyngeal insufficiency and phonatory change in up to 40–60% of patients [9, 10]. Severe complications are uncommon. *Reduction in the rate of complications likely reflects refinement in surgical technique*, with higher adverse events reported in studies published during the 1980s and lower frequencies in more recent decades [11]. Kezirian [12] published data on a large cohort of 3130 patients and reported mortality in 0.2% of patients and serious perioperative complications in 1.5%, results reproduced in other long-term studies [13, 14].

Early research was limited by the lack of high level trials, small numbers within trials, heterogeneity of the study groups and lack of consensus on what constituted surgical "success". However, whilst these limitations are still challenging in sleep surgery literature, emerging evidence suggests that outcomes with modified UPPP may provide similar outcomes to CPAP in quality of life and mortality domains [15, 16]. The SKUP [17] trial randomized 65 consecutive patients with moderate to severe OSA into two groups: the surgical arm underwent UPPP variant surgery, and the control group had limited conservative management for 7 months. Both groups had AHI and other PSG parameters compared at baseline and at the end of the study. There was a mean reduction in AHI of 60% in the UPPP group compared with an 11% reduction in AHI in the control group, a highly significant and clinically relevant finding. Follow-up studies demonstrated improvement in daytime sleepiness, vigilance and quality of life [18]. Another randomized controlled trial (RCT) [19] of 42 patients with moderate to severe OSA who had failed CPAP comprised two groups: the surgical arm underwent UPPP, and the control group did not receive treatment. In the surgical arm, 97% of patients were satisfied with the outcome, there was a mean reduction in AHI of 54% (compared with 12% in the control group) and there was also improvement in snoring and daytime somnolence.

Contemporary modifications of uvulopalatoplasty involve opening of the superolateral velopharyngeal ports without resection of functional soft tissue. One such technique is demonstrated in Fig. 5.1 [20].

In this technique, superolateral ports are opened by accessing and removing lateral palatal space fat [21]. The lateral palatal space is bounded medially by the curving fibres of palatopharyngeus muscle, laterally by the superior constrictor muscle, inferiorly by the superior pole of the tonsil, medially and ventrally by the palatoglossus muscle and ventrally by the mucosa of the palate. After removal of fat in this space, tension on the palatal folds is eliminated by a relatively high division of the posterior pillar and muscle complex. The proximal part of the musculo-mucosal complex is then repositioned by suturing it to the soft tissue adjacent to the space created by fat removal, sometimes as high as the tensor veli palatini fascia at the hamulus.

Variations on this technique are well described. Cahali [22] outlined the importance of the muscular lateral pharyngeal wall in the pathogenesis of OSA and was the first to develop a technique designed to splint the lateral pharyngeal wall. Li [23] developed the Taiwanese relocation pharyngoplasty, involving advancement of the soft palate and splinting of the lateral pharyngeal wall.

Other authors, such as Woodson and Pang [24], describe patient-specific modifications according to individual anatomy and include repositioning of the lateral wall of the pharynx and closure of the palatal pillars after tonsillectomy in what is

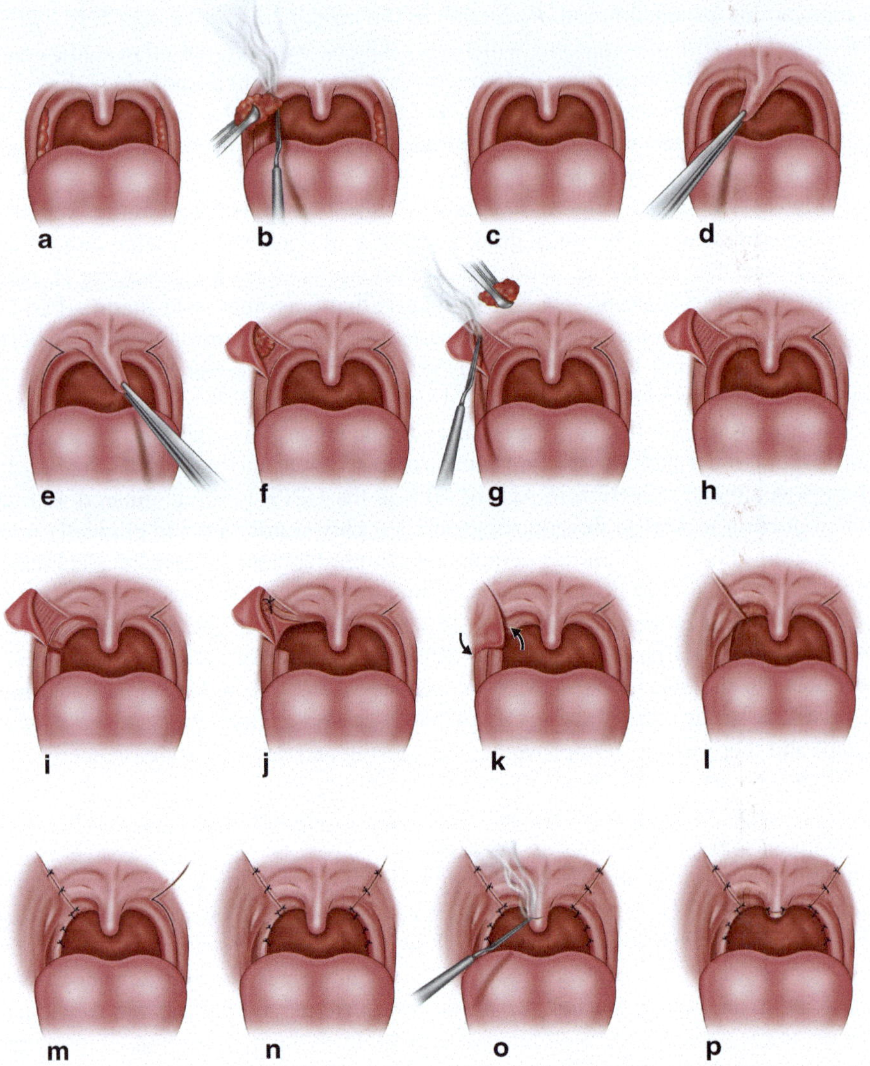

Fig. 5.1 Australian modified uvulopalatopharyngoplasty. (1) Resection of the tonsils, with preservation of pillar mucosa (**a**–**c**). (2) Traction on the uvula caudally while elevating a triangular flap of mucosa on each side as shown diagrammatically (**d**–**f**). (3) Resection of supratonsillar fat bilaterally (**g**). Demonstrating post-resection of supratonsillar fat (**h**). (4) Division of posterior pillar mucosa and musculature at the junction of upper third/lower two-thirds (**i**). (5) Suture advancement of the upper part of the posterior pillar musculature into the superolateral velopharyngeal port created in steps 2 and 3 using 2/0 Vicryl (**j**). (6) Closure of the overlying mucosa using 3/0 Vicryl (**k**–**n**). (7) Resection of approximately 50–75% of the uvula in a beveled fashion to create a neo-uvula (**o**, **p**)

referred to in the literature as expansion sphincteroplasty. The Woodson technique was adapted from Orticochea [25] and involves isolating the palatopharyngeus muscle, the main bulk of the lateral pharyngeal wall musculature, before rotating and repositioning this muscle to create lateral wall tension.

5.3.2 Tonsillectomy

The role of tonsillectomy alone in adults with OSA was the subject of a recent meta-analysis by Camacho et al. [26]. Seventeen studies were included for analysis. Success was defined as AHI <20/h and ≥50% reduction in AHI. This was achieved in over 85% of patients, with 57% achieving complete cure, defined as post-tonsillectomy AHI <5. Preoperative predictors of success included patients with large tonsils and AHI <30/h; therefore carefully selected patients for bilateral tonsillectomy alone is the key.

5.3.3 Resective/Ablative Techniques

The earliest techniques involved resection of the uvula and soft palate tissue [27]. Kamami [28] described laser-assisted uvulopalatoplasty (LAUP), an in-office procedure, with the patient in a seated position and performed under local anaesthesia. Its introduction was based on encouraging but limited short-term data [29]. Camacho [30] published a recent meta-analysis of longer-term data demonstrating poor success rates in OSA and worsening of the RDI or AHI in 44% of patients and concluded that the **LAUP be performed with caution or, preferably, not at all**. The provision of LAUP in Australia has had a marked decline in relative and absolute numbers [31], reflecting contemporary opinion that LAUP should be abandoned.

5.3.4 Stiffening Procedures

Pillar implants are designed to stiffen the palatal tissue involved in snoring to prevent vibration during breathing by inducing a local inflammatory response that creates fibrosis. Several studies [32–36] have assessed clinical effectiveness and efficacy, including one randomized, double-blind, sham surgery controlled trial by Friedman [37]. Overall, the authors of these studies reported significant but modest improvements in AHI in the context of mild OSA [35] and a reduction in snoring intensity and frequency [33, 34]. The technique is reportedly attractive for patients not willing to undergo traditional surgical correction [33]. However there is a risk of implant extrusion or awareness of the implant, with complication rates as high as 20%, particularly in women and those who undergo the procedure under general anaesthesia [37].

Other techniques, such as suturing, injection and radio frequency, designed to stiffen the soft palate, have been reported, and techniques continue to evolve. However, whilst these procedures are reported to be low-risk in-office procedures, it is not clear how effective they are in the long term. In a 6-year follow-up study on radio frequency of the soft palate for SDB [38], relapse of snoring was seen in nearly all of the 97% (74/77) of patients. Application of sutures to the soft palate to shorten, conglomerate and tense the tissue has been described, such as by Hur in 2008 [39], and also more recent variations in type and technique [40–42]. Injection snoreplasty involves a sclerosant directly infiltrated into the submucosal layer of the soft palate [43, 44]. Brietzke [45] reported reduction in subjective snoring "success rates" from 92 to 75% at a mean of 19-month follow-up.

5.3.5 Transpalatal Advancement

Transpalatal advancement (TPA) was described by Woodson in 1993 [46]. It is an adjunct to (modified) UPPP with the goal of increasing the volume of the velopharynx by removing the bone of the hard palate to facilitate fixation of the soft palate in an anterior position.

Two main incisional approaches to the hard palate bone have been described: the gothic arch incision [46] and the propeller incision [47]. Both give broad exposure to the hard palate, and the mucosal flaps raised are then elevated posteriorly over the palatine aponeurosis. The bone of the posterior part of the hard palate is then removed. The original description outlined removal of the entire posterior part of the hard palate, detaching the soft tissue from the bone centrally. A further modification was described, where a 2–3 mm strip of bone remained posteriorly, creating a bone island. Palate bone anterior to this is removed to create space into which the remaining island of tissue is advanced [46]. Division of the tensor veli palatini tendon laterally and pre-levator fascial fibres medially allows this tissue to be mobilized. The bone is secured with sutures passed through the anterior hard palate and back around the bone and soft tissue advancement flap. The mucosal flaps are approximated.

The cleft palate literature provides insights into palatal bone healing [48]. Understanding the factors contributing to healing is crucial because of the small but clinically significant risk of oronasal fistula. A robust soft tissue flap may allow the underlying bony anastomosis to heal, and, conversely, a poor soft tissue flap may compromise healing and result in oronasal fistula. Shine and Lewis reported a difference in flap survival between the traditional Gothic arch and the propeller incisions [47], and prevailing opinion holds that different flaps may be chosen for different arch heights of the palate. A recent systematic review and meta-analysis [49] examined the clinical efficacy of TPA in terms of AHI and lowest oxygen saturation. In the review, studies were excluded if concurrent surgeries for other levels of obstruction were performed at the same time. AHI and lowest oxygen saturation were improved with TPA: AHI reduced from 54.6 ± 23 preoperatively to 19.2 ± 16.8 postoperatively, and lowest oxygen saturation improved from 81.9 ± 8.1 preoperatively to 85.4 ± 6.9 postoperatively. Others, in concurrent surgical procedures excluded from analysis, have used this as a common component of multilevel airway surgery [50, 51].

5.4 Postoperative Complications

Common occurrences after palatal surgery in OSA include pain (usually managed with regular acetaminophen-based analgesia and other breakthrough pain relievers and steroids) and bleeding (similar incidence to tonsillectomy, when included with palatal surgery). In addition, procedure specific complications such as velopalatal insufficiency or VPI have a documented transient incidence—it occurs permanently only **very rarely** outside of the setting of "old style" ablative surgeries or revision operations. Oronasal fistula is the main operation specific concern in transpalatal advancement, and has been discussed by Shine and Lewis [47]. Management is usually conservative and includes dental-made temporary upper plate and rarely surgical closure.

In the Kezirian cohort [12], the authors identified three main risk factors for complications. These were increased body mass index (BMI), OSA severity (in that study, denoted by higher AHI) and comorbid disease. Other factors to consider are age and bleeding dyscrasias.

5.5 Future Directions and Summary

Despite the difficulties in running RCTs [52] and synthesizing the data into recommendations which can be applied to real-world practice, the application of future surgical therapies will need to be guided by high-level evidence. This will allow stratification of patients according to their individual anatomy and physiology and provide the basis for patient education. Within the next year, data form the Australian RCT comparing modified UPPP and coblation (radiofrequency in saline medium) tongue channeling with conservative treatment following device failure, will be available.

Currently the evidence supports a measured approach, incorporating careful patient and procedure selection and implementation of reconstructive palatal techniques, in order to achieve desirable outcomes in symptom and disease control.

References

1. Ikematsu T. Study of snoring, 4th report: therapy. J Jpn Otorhinolaryngol. 1964;64:434–5.
2. Fujita S, Conway W, Zorick F, Roth T. Surgical correction of anatomic abnormalities in obstructive sleep apnea syndrome: uvulopalatopharyngoplasty. Otolaryngol Head Neck Surg. 1981;89:923–34.
3. Sullivan CE, Issa FG, Berthon Jones M, Eves L. Reversal of obstructive sleep apnoea by continuous positive airway pressure applied through the nares. Lancet. 1981;317(8225):862–5.
4. Friedman M, Ibrahim H, Bass L. Clinical staging for sleep-disordered breathing. Otolaryngol Head Neck Surg. 2002;127:13–21.
5. Mallampati SR. Clinical sign to predict difficult tracheal intubation (hypothesis). Can Anaesth Soc J. 1983;30(3 Pt 1):316–7.
6. Eckert DJ, Malhotra A. Pathophysiology of adult obstructive sleep apnea. Proc Am Thorac Soc. 2008;5:144–53.

7. Joosten SA, Leong P, Landry SA, Sands SA, Terrill PI, Mann D, Turton A, Rangaswamy J, Andara C, Burgess G, Mansfield D, Hamilton GS, Edwards BA. Loop gain predicts the response to upper airway surgery in patients with obstructive sleep apnea. Sleep. 2017;40(7).
8. Holty JE, Guilleminault C. Surgical options for the treatment of obstructive sleep apnea. Med Clin North Am. 2010;94(3):479–515.
9. Grøntved AM, Karup P. Complaints and satisfaction after uvulopalatopharyngoplasty. Acta Otolaryngol. 2000;543:190–2.
10. Hagert B, Wikblad K, Odkvist L, Wahren LK. Side effects after surgical treatment of snoring. ORL J Otorhinolaryngol Relat Spec. 2000;62:76–80.
11. Franklin KA, Anttila H, Axelsson S, Gislason T, Maasilta P, Myhre KI, Rehnqvist N. Effects and side-effects of surgery for snoring and obstructive sleep apnea—a systematic review. Sleep. 2009;32(1):27–36.
12. Kezirian EJ, Weaver EM, Yueh B, Deyo RA, Khuri SF, Daley J, Henderson W. Incidence of serious complications after uvulopalatopharyngoplasty. Laryngoscope. 2004;114:450–3.
13. Marti S, Sampol G, Munoz X, et al. Mortality in severe sleep apnoea/hypopnoea syndrome patients: impact of treatment. Eur Respir J. 2002;20:1511–8.
14. Lin SH, Chen NH, Li HY, Fang TJ, Huang CC, Tsai YH. A comparison of the long-term outcome and effects of surgery or continuous positive airway pressure on patients with obstructive sleep apnea syndrome. Laryngoscope. 2006;116:1012–6.
15. Woods CM, Gunawardena I, Chia M, Vowles NJ, Ullah S, Robinson S, Carney AS. Long-term quality-of-life outcomes following treatment for adult obstructive sleep apnoea: comparison of upper airway surgery, continuous positive airway pressure and mandibular advancement splints. Clin Otolaryngol. 2016;41(6):762–70.
16. Weaver EM, Maynard C, Yueh B. Survival of veterans with sleep apnea: continuous positive airway pressure versus surgery. Otolaryngol Head Neck Surg. 2004;130:659–65.
17. Browaldh N, Nerfeldt P, Lysdahl M, Bring J, Friberg D. SKUP3 randomised controlled trial: polysomnographic results after uvulopalatopharyngoplasty in selected patients with obstructive sleep apnoea. Thorax. 2013;68:846–53.
18. Browaldh N, Bring J, Friberg D. SKUP(3) RCT; continuous study: changes in sleepiness and quality of life after modified UPPP. Laryngoscope. 2016;126(6):1484–91.
19. Sommer JU, Heiser C, Gahleitner C, Herr RM, Hörmann K, Maurer JT, Stuck BA. Tonsillectomy with uvulopalatopharyngoplasty in obstructive sleep apnea—a two-center randomized controlled trial. Dtsch Arztebl Int. 2016;113:1–8.
20. MacKay SG, Carney AS, Woods C, Antic N, McEvoy RD, Chia M, Sands T, Jones A, Hobson J, Robinson S. Modified uvulopalatopharyngoplasty and coblation channeling of the tongue for obstructive sleep apnea: a multi-centre Australian trial. J Clin Sleep Med. 2013;9:117–24.
21. Woodson BT, Tadokoro KS, MacKay SG. Radiofrequency ablation of the lateral palatal space for snoring. World J Otorhinolaryngol Head Neck Surg. 2017;3:106–9.
22. Cahali MB. Lateral pharyngoplasty: a new treatment for obstructive sleep apnea hypopnea syndrome. Laryngoscope. 2003;113(11):1961–8.
23. Li HY, Lee LA. Relocation pharyngoplasty for obstructive sleep apnea. Laryngoscope. 2009;119(12):2472–7.
24. Pang KP, Woodson BT. Expansion sphincter pharyngoplasty: a new technique for the treatment of obstructive sleep apnea. Otolaryngol Head Neck Surg. 2007;137(1):110–4.
25. Orticochea M. Construction of a dynamic muscle sphincter in cleft palates. Plast Reconstr Surg. 1968;41:323–7.
26. Camacho M, Li D, Kawai M, Zaghi S, Teixeira J, Senchak AJ, Brietzke SE, Frasier S, Certal V. Tonsillectomy for adult obstructive sleep apnea: a systematic review and meta-analysis. Laryngoscope. 2016;126(9):2176–86.
27. Heinberg CJ. A surgical procedure for the relief of snoring. Eye Ear Nose Throat Mon. 1955;34(6):389.
28. Kamami YV. Laser CO_2 for snoring. Preliminary results. Acta Otorhinolaryngol Belg. 1990;44(4):451–6.
29. Ryan CF. Laser assisted uvulopalatoplasty in sleep disordered breathing. Thorax. 1997;52:5–8.

30. Camacho M, Nesbitt NB, Lambert E, et al. Laser-assisted uvulopalatoplasty for obstructive sleep apnea: a systematic review and meta-analysis. Sleep. 2017;40(3).
31. Marshall N, MacKay S, Gallagher R, Robinson S. Uvulopalatopharyngoplasty funded by the Australian government's Medicare scheme (1995–2007). Otolaryngol Head Neck Surg. 2010;142:S10–4.
32. Choi JH, Cho JH, Chung YS, Kim JW, Kim SW. Effect of the pillar implant on snoring and mild obstructive sleep apnea: a multicenter study in Korea. Laryngoscope. 2015;125(5):1239–43.
33. Ho WK, Wei WI, Chung KF. Managing disturbing snoring with palatal implants: a pilot study. Arch Otolaryngol Head Neck Surg. 2004;130:753–8.
34. Lin HC, Friedman M, Chang HW, Lan CC, Chin CH, Lin MC, Pott T, Samuelson C. Effects of pillar implants for sleep-related breathing disorders on middle ear function. Eur Arch Otorhinolaryngol. 2013;270:2 339–2343.
35. Server EA, Alkan Z, Yiğit Ö, Yasak AG. Long-term results of pillar implant procedure. Kulak Burun Bogaz Ihtis Derg. 2016;26(5):258–64.
36. Gillespie MB, Smith JE, Clarke J, Nguyen SA. Effectiveness of pillar palatal implants for snoring management. Otolaryngol Head Neck Surg. 2009;140(3):363–8.
37. Friedman M, Schalch P, Lin HC, Kakodkar KA, Joseph NJ, Mazloom N. Palatal implants for the treatment of snoring and obstructive sleep apnea/hypopnea syndrome. Otolaryngol Head Neck Surg. 2008;138:209–16.
38. De Kermadec H, Blumen MB, Engalenc D, Vezina JP, Chabolle F. Radiofrequency of the soft palate for sleep-disordered breathing: a 6-year follow-up study. Eur Ann Otorhinolaryngol Head Neck Dis. 2014;131(1):27–31.
39. Hur J. A new treatment for snoring: sling snoreplasty with a permanent thread. Acta Otolaryngol. 2008;128(12):1381–4.
40. Murphey AW, Nguyen SA, Fuller C, Weber AC, Camilon MP, Gillespie MB. TranQuill sling snoreplasty for snoring: a single-arm pilot study for safety and effectiveness. Laryngoscope. 2016;126(1):243–8.
41. Mantovani M, Minetti A, Torretta S, Pincherle A, Tassone G, Pignatoro L. The velo-uvulo-pharyngeal lift or "roman blinds" technique for treatment of snoring: a preliminary report. Acta Otorhinolaryngol Ital. 2012;32:48–53.
42. Vicini C, Hendaway E, Campanini A. Barbed reposition pharyngoplasty (BRP) for OSAHS: a feasibility, safety, efficacy and teachability pilot study. "We are on the giant's shoulders". Eur Arch Otorhinolaryngol. 2015;272:3065–70.
43. Brietze SE, Mair EA. Injection snoreplasty: how to treat snoring without all the pain and expense. Otolaryngol Head Neck Surg. 2001;124(5):503–10.
44. Straus JF. A new approach to the treatment of snoring. Arch Otolaryngol. 1943;38:225–9.
45. Brietzke SE, Mair EA. Injection snoreplasty: extended follow-up and new objective data. Otolaryngol Head Neck Surg. 2003;128(5):605–15.
46. Woodson BT, Toohill RJ. Transpalatal advancement pharyngoplasty for obstructive sleep apnea. Laryngoscope. 1993;103:269–76.
47. Shine NP, Lewis RH. The "propeller" incision for transpalatal advancement pharyngoplasty: a new approach to reduce post-operative oronasal fistulae. Auris Nasus Larynx. 2008;35:397–400.
48. Yin N, Ma L, Zhang Z. Bone regeneration in the hard palate after cleft palate surgery. Plast Reconstr Surg. 2005;115(5):1239–44.
49. Volner K, Dunn B, Chang ET, Song SA, Liu SYC, Brietzke SE, O'Connor P, Camacho M. Transpalatal advancement pharyngoplasty for obstructive sleep apnea: a systematic review and meta-analysis. Eur Arch Otorhinolaryngol. 2017;274:1197–203.
50. MacKay SG, Jefferson N, Grundy L, Lewis R. Coblation-assisted Lewis and MacKay operation (CobLAMO): new technique for tongue reduction in sleep apnoea surgery. J Laryngol Otol. 2013;127(12):1222–5.
51. Robinson S, Chia M, Carney AS, Chawla S, Harris P, Esterman A. Upper airway reconstructive surgery long-term quality-of-life outcomes compared with CPAP for adult obstructive sleep apnea. Otolaryngol Head Neck Surg. 2009;141(2):257–63.
52. MacKay SG, Chan L. Surgical approaches to obstructive sleep apnea. Sleep Med Clin. 2016;11(3):331–41.

Base of Tongue Surgery

6

Claudio Vicini, Filippo Montevecchi, Giuseppe Meccariello, and Giovanni Cammaroto

6.1 Introduction

The gold standard treatment for OSAHS is usually considered continuous positive airway pressure (CPAP). However, a variable but significant number of patients are not able to tolerate this device and require an alternative treatment. Surgery is one of the possible alternative options, even if it has been criticized due to a lack of evidence to support its efficacy as well as the heterogencous reporting of published outcomes. The most commonly reported surgical procedure is, without any doubt, uvulopalatopharyngoplasty (UPPP). However, considering the frequent multilevel obstruction highlighted by means of sleep endoscopy [1], treatment of lingual obstruction has become more popular.

Coblation tongue surgery and, more recently, trans-oral robotic surgery (TORS) proved to be the most published therapeutic options in the area of the tissue reduction techniques [2–4].

In the present chapter, we try to give an overview of the literature about the use of Coblation and TORS for the treatment of OSAHS in adults.

6.2 Review of Literature

An overview on the surgical techniques that can be performed adopting these two technologies is given in this chapter. From the analysis of recent literature, only posterior midline glossectomy and lingual tonsillectomy were reported to be used both with Coblation and robotic support.

C. Vicini · F. Montevecchi (✉) · G. Meccariello · G. Cammaroto
Head and Neck Department, ENT and Oral Surgery Unit, G.B. Morgagni—L. Pierantoni Hospital, Forlì, Infermi Hospital, Faenza, ASL of Romagna, Italy
e-mail: claudio@claudiovicini.com

S. O. Salman (ed.), *Modern Management of Obstructive Sleep Apnea*,
https://doi.org/10.1007/978-3-030-11443-5_6

Fifteen articles (seven for TORS, seven for Coblation and one reporting on both technologies) were analysed [5–19] following these inclusion criteria: (1) available information on outcome data; (2) data concerning the type of surgical treatment (exclusive robotic/Coblation surgery, associated with palatal/nose surgery, previous surgical treatment); and (3) data regarding the preoperative and postoperative values of apnea-hypopnea index (AHI), body mass index (BMI), lowest saturation of peripheral oxygen (SpO2), Epworth sleepiness scale (ESS), hospital stay, complications, starting of oral feeding and need for tracheostomy.

The mean of enrolled patients for TORS was 102.5 comprising a total of 820 cases. The mean age was 49, and 285 patients (34.7%) underwent a previous sleep apnea surgery which consisted of nasal surgery in the most of cases.

The mean of enrolled patients for Coblation was 32.7 comprising a total of 262 cases. The mean age of the evaluated patents was 42.5, and 40 patients (15.3%) underwent a previous sleep apnea surgery which consisted of palatal surgery in all cases.

Palatal surgery was performed simultaneously in 37.4% of patients treated with TORS, with UPPP being the most common procedure (71.3%), followed by expansion sphincter pharyngoplasty (ESP) (15.3%). Epiglottoplasty was performed in association with robotic tongue base reduction in 48.5% of cases. Few patients ($n = 5$) underwent a tracheostomy: four preventive tracheostomies and one urgent procedure after lingual bleeding.

Palatal surgery was performed in 83.5% of patients treated with Coblation, with UPPP being the most common procedure (56.7%), followed by Z-plasty (33.8%). Epiglottoplasty and tracheostomy were never performed in association with Coblation.

The mean rates of failure were 34.4% and 38.5%, respectively, in TORS and Coblation groups.

Complications occurred in 21.3% of the patients treated with TORS ($n = 820$). Transient dysphagia represented the most common complication (7.2%) followed by bleeding (4.2%). Minor complications such as postoperative pharyngeal oedema were registered in 1% of cases. Least reported events were transient dysgeusia, transient dysphagia and globus.

Complications occurred in 8.4% of the patients treated with Coblation surgery ($n = 262$). Bleeding represented the most common complication (2.6%) followed by postoperative oedema (2.2%) and globus (1.1%). Least reported events were transient dysgeusia and hypoglossus injury.

6.3 Discussion

The surgical treatment of OSAHS is registering an increasing popularity for many reasons, including the development of new technologies such as Coblation and TORS.

The first paper about Tongue Base Coblation was presented to scientific community as a therapeutic tool for sleep disorders in 2005 [3].

The first paper pioneering the use of TORS in OSAHS patients was published by Vicini et al. in 2010 [2]. Recently, researchers seem to have focused their attention more on TORS, with a significant peak in the publication of papers registered in 2015. On the other hand, the trend for Coblation is downward, with a consistent reduction of the scientific production seen from 2013 to 2014. This trend probably reflects the relative delay between the launch of Coblation some years before the more recent introduction of TORS.

All evaluated papers except one are retrospective, and a well-designed prospective study is so far missing in the worldwide literature. In most of the reported series, the number of cases is sufficient but not really large.

Coblation for the treatment of the hypertrophy of the base of the tongue in patients affected by OSAHS seems to be especially popular in Asia and, in particular, widespread as a therapeutic option for young patients [20]. This technology has been mostly presented by the Chinese scientific community with a significant lack of English language papers.

Friedman et al. published the only comparative study between the two technologies in 2012. However, the two surgical techniques performed adopting Coblation and TORS were not completely comparable, being a posterior midline glossectomy and a submucosal minimally invasive lingual excision, respectively. The authors highlighted that patients undergoing robot-assisted surgery took longer to tolerate normal diet and to resume normal activity, even though the most significant reduction of AHI was seen in patients treated with TORS. On the other hand, Friedman underlined that procedural costs and operating room time were increased with the robotic technique. In particular, disposable costs were $730 per robotic procedure and $250 per Coblation procedure [5].

Taking into consideration the different sizes of the two groups (TORS = 820 vs Coblation = 262), the following can be stated. Epiglottoplasty was never performed in patients treated with Coblation, while it was included in almost half of the patients undergoing a TORS surgery. This data may also explain the slightly better PSG outcomes obtained in TORS patients. In fact, from the last systematic review by Torre et al., it seems that the prevalence of epiglottis collapse in OSAHS is greater than previously reported. For this reason, drug-induced sleep endoscopy (DISE) may play a pivotal role in the understanding of OSAHS pathogenesis addressing physicians to choose epiglottoplasty when needed [21].

Clinical and polysomnography improvement seemed not to be significantly different between the two groups, even though a lower rate of failure was registered in TORS patients (TORS = 34.3% vs Coblation = 38.5%). This slight difference between the two surgical options may however be more consistent considering that a higher percentage of patients treated with TORS had previously undergone a surgical procedure for OSAHS (TORS = 34.7% vs Coblation = 15.3%) and preoperative AHI and BMI values were higher in TORS group.

Conversely, complication rates were consistently lower in patients treated with Coblation surgery. However, major complications such as intraoperative and postoperative bleedings were infrequent in both groups.

From a careful analysis of the literature, it can be observed that Coblation and robotic technologies support several different surgical techniques. In our opinion, this is a key point in the critical comparison of Coblation versus TORS. Strictly speaking, Coblation is an advanced, low-temperature, relatively cheap, cutting technology, requiring a separate and independent set of very different tools for exposing, visualizing and manipulating the surgical area (e.g. headlamp, loupe glasses, handheld or self-retaining 2D video endoscope). On the other hand, TORS by da Vinci platform is a very high-tech and expensive technology offering superb 3D vision and a very precise computer-assisted "enhanced" tele-manipulation, requiring some additional cutting device such as monopolar or laser according to the surgeon's preference (Fig. 6.1). Both technologies may be used in a wide latitude of surgical techniques, different for extension and geometry of resection in surface and depth, for different ratio between lymphoid/muscular tissue removed, for a transmucosal vs submucosal resection and for different additional procedures associated to base of tongue surgery in the supraglottic region, palate, palatine tonsils, adenoids, nose and paranasal sinuses.

However, there are some other factors that should be taken into consideration.

In particular, TORS surgery supports a 3–5 hand technique, while no more than three hands can be used in Coblation procedures (Fig. 6.2). Moreover, the resection of a measurable portion of tongue seems to be another advantage of TORS surgery.

After an overview of the different surgical techniques reported in literature, we may summarize the following list of different surgical techniques.

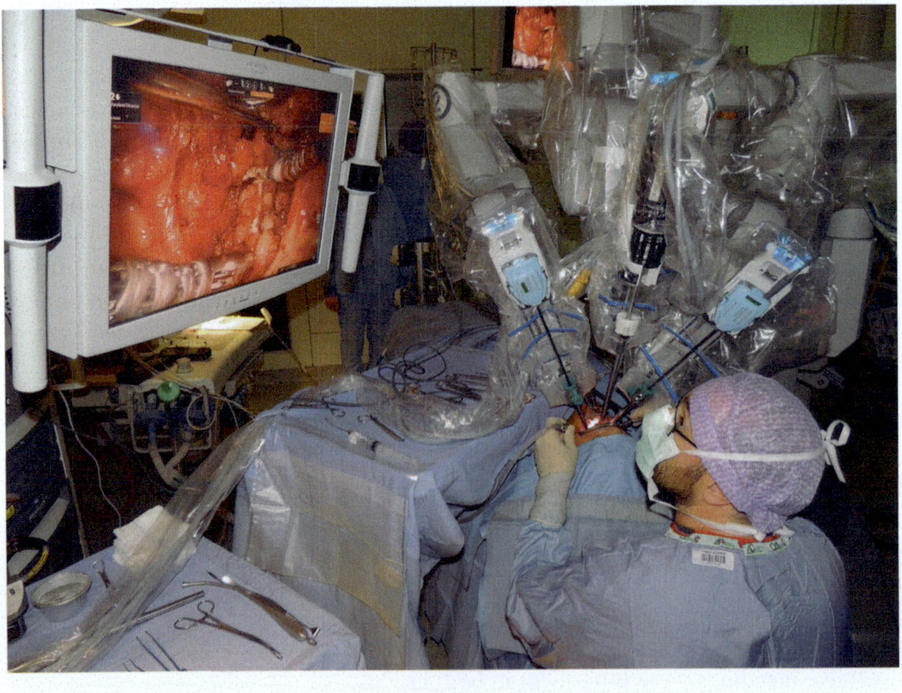

Fig. 6.1 Operating room during TORS. The bedside assistant can follow all the surgical steps on the monitor while the first surgeon is working at the robotic console

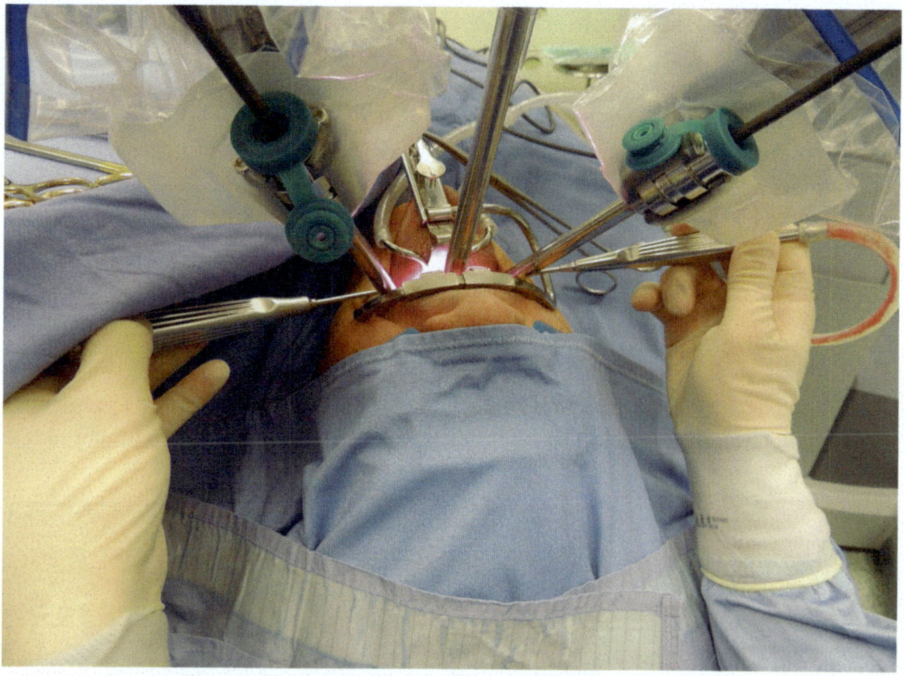

Fig. 6.2 Robotic surgical field. The advantage of robotic surgery is the possibility to work inside the oropharynx with five hands (three robotic arms for instruments and scope and two instruments handled by the assistant, usually suctions or bipolar)

6.4 Surgical Procedures Overview

6.4.1 Lingual Tonsillectomies

The common trait of this group of procedures is the selective removal of hypertrophic lymphoid tissue, without any violation of the underlying muscle. Generally speaking this technique is quick, easy and safe (lymphoid tissue doesn't include critical vessels and/or nerves). This group of procedures is limited to cases of significant lingual tonsil hypertrophy as exclusive obstructing pathology. On the contrary, the other techniques may be indicated in any kind of muscular tongue obstruction.

6.4.2 Posterior Midline Glossectomies

A variable amount of lymphoid tissue and muscle is resected around the midline, with different possible shape in section: "V" or "U" shape or "Δ" shape. The rationale of a midline muscle removal is the aim of work inside a central safe corridor far from vessel and nerves. A careful dissection under magnification may allow the identification and conservation of vessel and nerves if encountered. Besides the tongue volume reduction, an additional airway clearance may arise from the final scalloping in the midline.

6.4.3 Tongue Base Reduction With/Without Supraglottoplasties

A composite (lymphoid tissue and muscle) layer of tongue base is progressively removed, deeper around the midline, with a final "T" or "mushroom" shape in section. A careful dissection under magnification may allow the identification and conservation of vessel and nerves if encountered. The rationale of this solution is to optimize the tissue removed volume, working in superficial and deep safe areas, with the final result of more tissue dissected (Figs. 6.3, 6.4, 6.5, 6.6, 6.7, and 6.8).

6.4.4 Submucosal Glossectomies

Overemphasis on the concept of superficial covering conservation, in order to reduce pain and promote a quicker healing, it is possible to carry out a tunnel in the

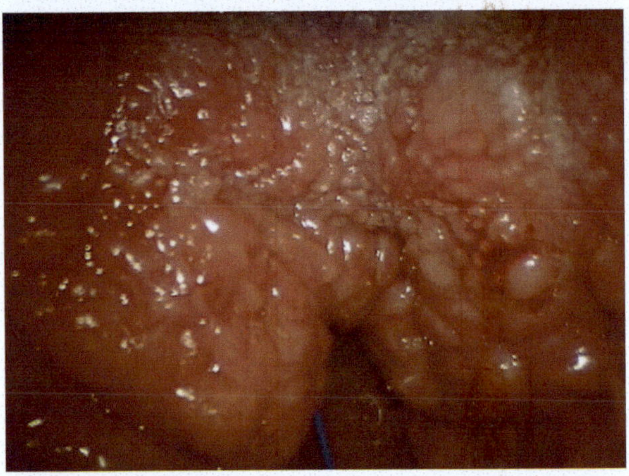

Fig. 6.3 Surgical field at the beginning of the procedure. Lymphatic hypertrophy of the tongue base posteriorly to the circumvallate papillae

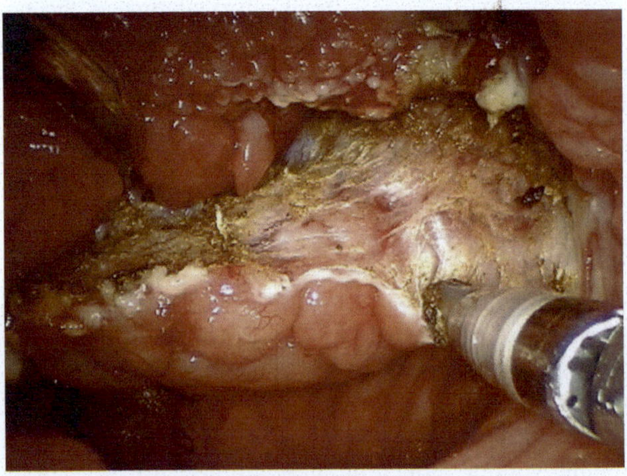

Fig. 6.4 Dissection of the right tongue base using a monopolar cautery and a Maryland forceps, 5 mm robotic instruments

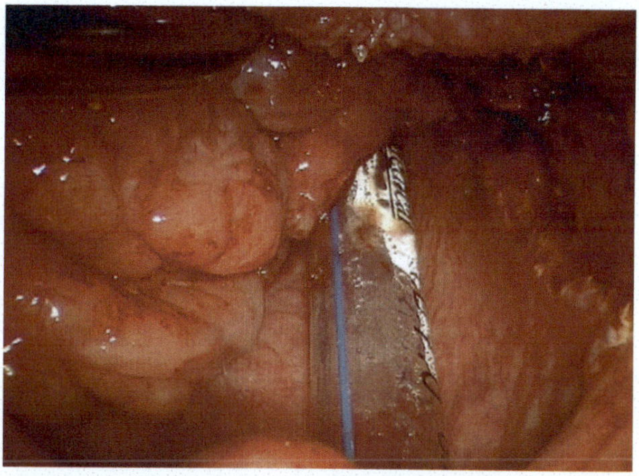

Fig. 6.5 Surgical field at the end of the right tongue base dissection

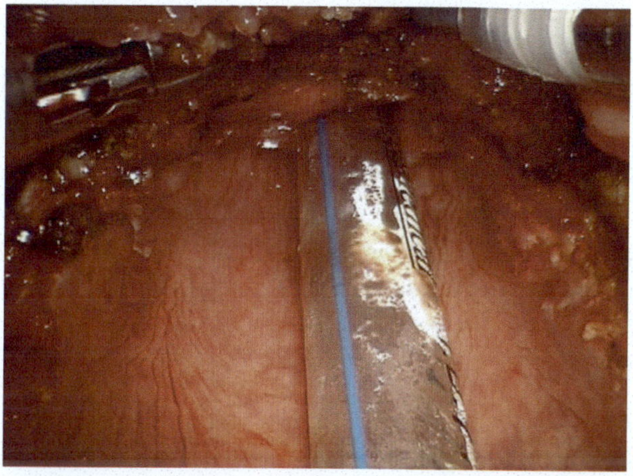

Fig. 6.6 Surgical field at the end of the left and right tongue base dissection

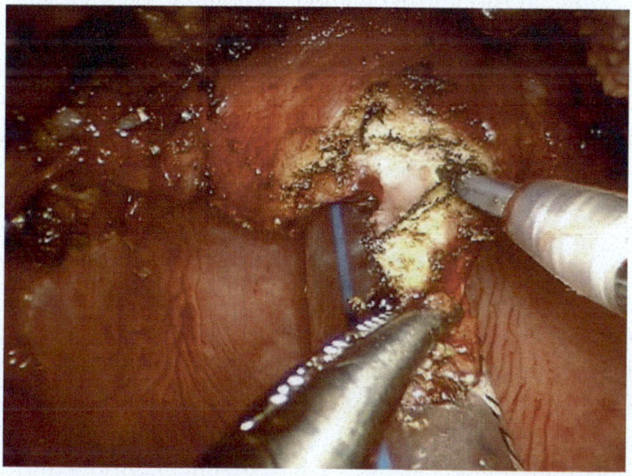

Fig. 6.7 Robotic epiglottoplasty

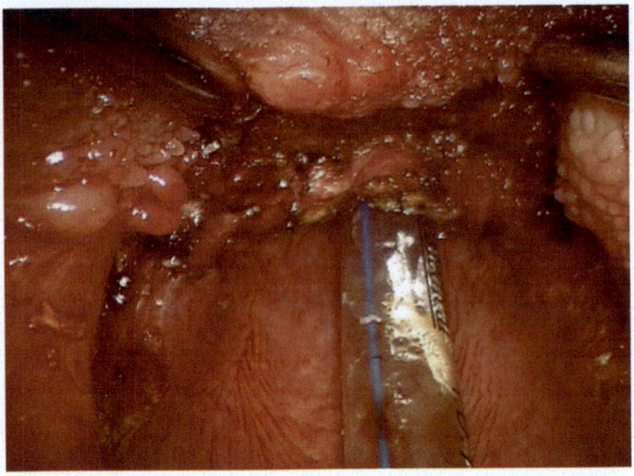

Fig. 6.8 Surgical field at the end of the procedure

midline of the tongue where the instrument can be inserted. An ultrasound mapping of lingual artery course is strongly recommended, and the progression of the dissection is controlled by digital palpation instead of direct visualization.

6.5 Summary

In particular, only posterior midline glossectomy and lingual tonsillectomy were reported to be performed with the use of both technologies. On the other hand, some surgical techniques such as tongue base reduction and submucosal glossectomies seem to be exclusively supported by TORS and Coblation, respectively.

In our opinion, it is useful to interpret the scientific literature taking the technical aspect into consideration. From a preliminary comparison of Lin, Friedman, Li and Wee's experiences, posterior midline glossectomy seems to have similar effectiveness in both groups. However, there are no studies comparing the same technique performed adopting Coblation and robotic surgery.

Another important aspect that may require surgeons' attention is postoperative pain. From some authors' experience, it seems that the use of Coblation in tonsillectomy reduces postoperative pain in comparison with monopolar electrocautery [22]. Despite the lack of literature, these results may be found also in patients undergoing a surgery of the base of tongue.

The last aspect that needs to be discussed regards the costs of both procedures. From our team's experience, the average cost of a patient who undergoes robotic surgery may range approximately between 4500 and 6000 euros (depending on the hospital stay). Considering Friedman's economic evaluation on the disposable tools, Coblation surgery may cost $500 less than TORS per patient [5], not considering that the purchase of a robotic system is significantly more expensive than Coblation (around $2,000,000 vs $20,000).

In conclusion, considering the evaluated outcomes and the lack of studies comparing the use of the same surgical techniques performed with TORS and Coblation, both technologies seem to be reliable. Moreover, a growing interest towards the use of these tools on the paediatric population has also been recently seen, with robotic or Coblation lingual tonsillectomy being the most common surgical procedure [23–25].

Finally, taking into consideration the low rate of major complications of the two therapeutic options, TORS seems to give slightly better results, allowing a wider surgical view and a more consistent removal of lingual tissue. However, the higher rate of minor complication and the significant costs of TORS must also be considered. The key point that must be overemphasized is that both technologies may be applied to a very wide range of surgical techniques, each of them presumably with different degrees of effectiveness.

References

1. Campanini A, Canzi P, De Vito A, Dallan I, Montevecchi F, Vicini C. Awake versus sleep endoscopy: personal experience in 250 OSAHS patients. Acta Otorhinolaryngol Ital. 2010;30(2):73–7.
2. Vicini C, Dallan I, Canzi P, Frassineti S, La Pietra MG, Montevecchi F. Transoral robotic tongue base resection in obstructive sleep apnoea-hypopnoea syndrome: a preliminary report. ORL J Otorhinolaryngol Relat Spec. 2010;72(1):22–7.
3. He M, Chen H, Jin W, He Y, Su Z, Fan Y, Yu C. Uvulopalatopharyngoplasty and tongue base coblation treat the 112 cases of severe obstructive sleep apnea-hypopnea syndrome. Lin Chuang Er Bi Yan Hou Ke Za Zhi. 2005;19(23):1061.
4. Cammaroto G, Montevecchi F, D'Agostino G, Zeccardo E, Bellini C, Galletti B, Shams M, Negm H, Vicini C. Tongue reduction for OSAHS: TORSs vs coblations, technologies vs techniques, apples vs oranges. Eur Arch Otorhinolaryngol. 2017;274(2):637–45.
5. Friedman M, Hamilton C, Samuelson CG, Kelley K, Taylor D, Pearson-Chauhan K, Maley A, Taylor R, Venkatesan TK. Transoral robotic glossectomy for the treatment of obstructive sleep apnea-hypopnea syndrome. Otolaryngol Head Neck Surg. 2012;146(5):854–62.
6. Hoff PT, D'Agostino MA, Thaler ER. Transoral robotic surgery in benign diseases including obstructive sleep apnea: safety and feasibility. Laryngoscope. 2015;125(5):1249–53.
7. Vicini C, Montevecchi F, Campanini A, Dallan I, Hoff PT, Spector ME, Thaler E, Ahn J, Baptista P, Remacle M, Lawson G, Benazzo M, Canzi P. Clinical outcomes and complications associated with TORS for OSAHS: a benchmark for evaluating an emerging surgical technology in a targeted application for benign disease. ORL J Otorhinolaryngol Relat Spec. 2014;76(2):63–9.
8. Toh ST, Han HJ, Tay HN, Kiong KL. Transoral robotic surgery for obstructive sleep apnea in Asian patients: a Singapore sleep centre experience. JAMA Otolaryngol Head Neck Surg. 2014;140(7):624–9.
9. Muderris T, Sevil E, Bercin S, Gul F, Kiris M. Transoral robotic lingual tonsillectomy in adults: preliminary results. Acta Otolaryngol. 2015;135(1):64–9.
10. Hoff PT, Glazer TA, Spector ME. Body mass index predicts success in patients undergoing transoral robotic surgery for obstructive sleep apnea. ORL J Otorhinolaryngol Relat Spec. 2014;76(5):266–72.
11. Lin HS, Rowley JA, Folbe AJ, Yoo GH, Badr MS, Chen W. Transoral robotic surgery for treatment of obstructive sleep apnea: factors predicting surgical response. Laryngoscope. 2015;125(4):1013–20.
12. Thaler ER, Rassekh CH, Lee JM, Weinstein GS, O'Malley BW Jr. Outcomes for multilevel surgery for sleep apnea: obstructive sleep apnea, transoral robotic surgery, and uvulopalatopharyngoplasty. Laryngoscope. 2016;126(1):266–9.

13. MacKay SG, Carney AS, Woods C, Antic N, McEvoy RD, Chia M, Sands T, Jones A, Hobson J, Robinson S. Modified uvulopalatopharyngoplasty and coblation channeling of the tongue for obstructive sleep apnea: a multi-centre Australian trial. J Clin Sleep Med. 2013;9(2):117–24.
14. Hou T, Hu S, Jiang X. Tongue coblation via the ventral approach for obstructive sleep apnea-hypopnea syndrome surgery. Laryngoscope. 2012;122(11):2582–6.
15. Wang L, Liu JX, Yang XL, Yang CW, Qin YX. Z-palatoplasty and tongue radiofrequency for patients with small tonsils. Otolaryngol Head Neck Surg. 2013;148(5):873–7.
16. Wee JH, Tan K, Lee WH, Rhee CS, Kim JW. Evaluation of coblation lingual tonsil removal technique for obstructive sleep apnea in Asians: preliminary results of surgical morbidity and prognosticators. Eur Arch Otorhinolaryngol. 2015;272(9):2327–33.
17. Li HY, Lee LA, Kezirian EJ. Coblation endoscopic lingual lightening (CELL) for obstructive sleep apnea. Eur Arch Otorhinolaryngol. 2016;273(1):231–6.
18. Babademez MA, Ciftci B, Acar B, Yurekli MF, Karabulut H, Yilmaz A, Karasen RM. Low-temperature bipolar radiofrequency ablation (coblation) of the tongue base for supine-position-associated obstructive sleep apnea. ORL J Otorhinolaryngol Relat Spec. 2010;72(1):51–5.
19. Friedman M, Soans R, Gurpinar B, Lin HC, Joseph N. Evaluation of submucosal minimally invasive lingual excision technique for treatment of obstructive sleep apnea/hypopnea syndrome. Otolaryngol Head Neck Surg. 2008;139(3):378–84; discussion 385.
20. Li D, Zhang Q, Song W. A retrospective study of 768 coblation treatment in children with obstructive sleep apnea-hypopnea syndrome. Lin Chung Er Bi Yan Hou Tou Jing Wai Ke Za Zhi. 2014;28(7):453–4, 458.
21. Torre C, Camacho M, Liu SY, Huon LK, Capasso R. Epiglottis collapse in adult obstructive sleep apnea: a systematic review. Laryngoscope. 2016;126(2):515–23.
22. Parker NP, Walner DL. Post-operative pain following coblation or monopolar electrocautery tonsillectomy in children: a prospective, single-blinded, randomised comparison. Clin Otolaryngol. 2011;36(5):468–74.
23. Thottam PJ, Govil N, Duvvuri U, Mehta D. Transoral robotic surgery for sleep apnea in children: is it effective? Int J Pediatr Otorhinolaryngol. 2015;79(12):2234–7.
24. Lin AC, Koltai PJ. Persistent pediatric obstructive sleep apnea and lingual tonsillectomy. Otolaryngol Head Neck Surg. 2009;141(1):81–5.
25. Maturo SC, Mair EA. Submucosal minimally invasive lingual excision: an effective, novel surgery for pediatric tongue base reduction. Ann Otol Rhinol Laryngol. 2006;115(8):624–30.

7 Upper Airway Stimulation

Jason L. Yu and Erica R. Thaler

7.1 Introduction

Surgical management of obstructive sleep apnea has been a method of treatment since Fujita first published his outcomes using uvulopalatopharyngoplasty to treat obstructive sleep apnea [1]. Since that time, surgical therapies have consisted of various types of ablative or repositioning surgeries. Surgical success of these techniques has been highly variable ranging from 35 to 95% [2–4].

Upper airway stimulation (UAS) is a novel approach for treatment of OSA. Unlike previous methods of surgical management of obstructive sleep apnea (OSA) that relies on static repositioning or ablation of soft tissue, UAS utilizes electrical stimulation to activate the intrinsic and extrinsic muscles of the tongue to open the pharynx. One benefit to patients is that there is no removal or alteration of patient's airway anatomy from this surgery. Stimulation also addresses a fundamental limitation of ablation and repositioning surgeries which is the change in muscular tone and dilator activity that accompanies OSA [5].

In 2014, the FDA approved Inspire, the first upper airway stimulation device, (Inspire Medical Systems, Minneapolis, MN) for treatment of obstructive sleep apnea [6]. Inspire consists of an implantable pulse generator (IPG) which is placed in a subcutaneous pocket on the chest with an electrode tunneled to the hypoglossal nerve and a pressure sensor tunneled into the intercostal muscles of the chest (Fig. 7.1). During inspiration, the pressure sensor triggers the IPG to generate an electrical stimulus to the hypoglossal nerve causing the tongue to protrude. Activation/deactivation of the device is controlled by the patient via a handheld remote. The STAR trial, the initial multicenter trial, showed an average AHI

J. L. Yu · E. R. Thaler (✉)
Department of Otolaryngology Head and Neck Surgery, Hospital of the University of Pennsylvania, Philadelphia, PA, USA
e-mail: Jason.yu2@uphs.upenn.edu; erica.thaler@uphs.upenn.edu

S. O. Salman (ed.), *Modern Management of Obstructive Sleep Apnea*,
https://doi.org/10.1007/978-3-030-11443-5_7

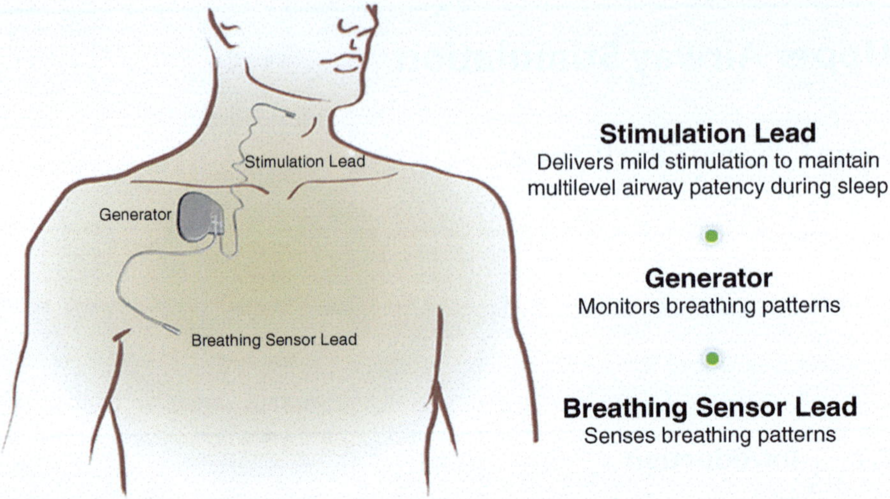

Fig. 7.1 Inspire device with implantable pulse generator connected to electrode and pressure sensor leads

reduction from 32.0 to 15.3 [6]. Subsequent 3 and 5 years' follow-up of patients since the original trial showed persistent durable response to therapy [7, 8].

Inspire is the first device introduced onto the market for the treatment of OSA using electrical stimulation of nerves to maintain upper airway tone. Its results have shown that upper airway stimulation is a viable way for management of OSA. Other devices are currently under investigation looking to use UAS as a means of treatment (ImThera Medical, San Diego, CA) [9]. Ultimately, UAS has proven to be an effective new method for the surgical management of OSA, and future studies will focus on the long-term outcomes of this modality of therapy.

7.2 Preoperative Evaluation

Patients being evaluated for upper airway stimulation should be evaluated by a dedicated sleep physician or surgeon. A comprehensive history and physical examination should be performed. A type 1 polysomnogram is required, and an apnea-hypopnea index (AHI) between 15 and 65 is necessary to qualify. There should be attempts to optimize noninvasive therapies including CPAP, BIPAP, and oral appliance therapy. It is also important to encourage lifestyle modifications including weight loss, optimizing sleep hygiene, and addressing medical comorbidities. Patients unable to maintain or unwilling to try first-line treatment should be considered for surgical intervention. The original STAR trial included patients with body mass index (BMI) less than 32; however, currently the upper limit per FDA stipulation is 35. It should be noted that successful implantations have occurred in patients with BMI >35 [10]. Patients must undergo diagnostic sleep endoscopy

(DISE) to assess for upper airway stimulation candidacy [11]. Assessment of retropalatal, retroglossal, and supraglottic regions should be assessed during DISE. Presence of anteroposterior collapse at the retropalatal region will qualify for UAS. Patients with concentric collapse at the retropalatal region were shown to be more likely to fail therapy and therefore should not receive UAS. Other contraindications listed by the company include:

- Central + mixed apneas >25% of the total apnea-hypopnea index.
- Any condition or procedure that has compromised neurological control of the upper airway.
- Patients who are unable or do not have the necessary assistance to operate the sleep remote.
- Patients who are pregnant or plan to become pregnant.
- Arc welders.
- Inspire Model 3024 is not MRI compatible but Model 3028 can under MRI on the head and extremities under certain conditions.

7.3 Surgical Technique

The procedure is performed under general anesthesia. Long-acting neuromuscular blockade should be avoided as neuromonitoring (i.e., NIM-Response 3.0 System, Medtronic Xomed, Jacksonville, Florida) is needed to help identify branches of the hypoglossal nerve. The head of the bed should be 180° from anesthesia to facilitate easy access to the head for lead placement and testing. Two sets of electrodes are placed within the tongue musculature for neuromonitoring. One set is placed in the floor of the mouth entering into the genioglossus muscle, the primary protruder of the tongue, and the second is placed along the ipsilateral lateral tongue into the hyoglossus and styloglossus muscles, retractors of the tongue. Perioperative antibiotics (e.g., 2 g cefazolin) for coverage of skin flora should be given at the onset of anesthesia. Skin should be prepped from the angle of the mandible down to the lower edge of the ribcage from the sternum to the posterior axilla. The surgery is typically performed on the right side, although left-sided implantation can be performed if medically required. Three incisions are made during the procedure, one under the mandible, one along the ipsilateral anterior chest, and one along the anterior axilla at the lower ribs.

The first incision is a 4-cm incision made in the ipsilateral upper neck 1–2 cm below the inferior border of the mandible and anterior to the submandibular gland to avoid the marginal mandibular nerve. Identification of the posterior edge of the anterior belly of the digastric is the first consistent landmark encountered. The muscle is then followed posteriorly to the digastric tendon. Palpation of the hyoid bone can also assist in locating the digastric tendon if exposure is difficult. The border between the anterior portion of the submandibular gland and the mylohyoid muscle can then be identified. The anterior portion of the hypoglossal nerve will lie deep to this muscle. Retraction of the anterior border of the submandibular gland posterosuperiorly and the mylohyoid muscle anteriorly will reveal the hypoglossal nerve. Once the main trunk is identified, it can be followed anteriorly until it begins to branch. Neurostimulation at this time can help identify branches to the genioglossus which should be included in the electrode placement for stimulation. Branches to the styloglossus and hyoglossus which are retractor muscles should not be included in electrode placement. The electrode cuff can be placed around the desired nerve branches (Fig. 7.2). The electrode wire is then tunneled under the digastric muscle and secured to its surface with two 3–0 silk sutures.

The second incision is placed along the ipsilateral chest about 3 cm inferior to the clavicle. Dissection through the subcutaneous fat until the fascia overlying the pectoralis muscle is seen. A pocket is made over the pectoralis fascia muscle for placement of the implantable pulse generator (IPG).

The third incision is made along the anterior mid-axillary line overlying the intercostal space between the fourth and sixth ribs. Blunt dissection down to the intercostal muscles is performed. A tunnel between the external and internal intercostal muscles is then made, and a malleable retractor is placed into the pocket to keep it open for placement of the sensor lead. The sensor lead is then placed into the pocket between the external and internal intercostal muscles. This is secured to the fascia of the chest using 3–0 silk sutures to attach two anchoring devices. Both the electrode and sensor lead are then tunneled subcutaneously from their respective sites into the chest incision to connect to the IPG. The IPG is then secured in the chest pocket using two 3–0 silk sutures.

Once the IPG is connected to both sensor and stimulation leads, initial testing is performed with measurements of respiratory effort and test stimulation with confirmation of tongue protrusion intraoperatively. A lateral neck and chest X-ray are obtained in the post-anesthesia care unit (PACU) to confirm proper placement of the leads and IPG and to rule out pneumothorax. The surgery is an outpatient procedure, and patients can be discharged the same day.

Patients follow up with the surgeon at 1 week for a wound check, and activation of the device occurs at 1 month to allow healing. Once activated, a titration sleep study is performed at 2 months to determine optimum voltage characterization of the device.

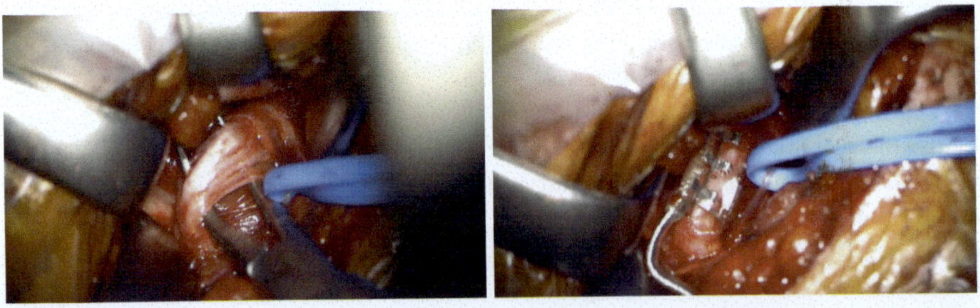

Fig. 7.2 Identification of the anterior branch of hypoglossal nerve and subsequent placement of the electrode. It is important to confirm stimulation of the genioglossus muscle with neurostimulation

7.4 Postoperative Complications

There are several possible adverse effects following surgery. These include:

- Damage to blood vessels in the vicinity of implant
- Excessive bleeding
- Nerve trauma or damage
- Allergic and/or rejection response to the implanted materials
- Infection
- Local irritation, seroma, hematoma, erosion, or swelling
- Persistent pain, numbness, or inflammation at the implant site
- Discomfort form the stimulation
- Tongue movement restrictions, irritation resulting from tongue abrasions on pre-existing sharp or broken teeth
- Tongue soreness or weakness
- Problems with swallowing or speaking
- Undesirable change in stimulation over time, possible related to tissue changes around electrodes, shifts in electrode position, loose electrical connections, or lead fractures
- Fibrosis to the extent that makes it difficult to remove the system without damaging surrounding structures
- Dry mouth
- Other acute symptoms (i.e., headaches, coughing, choking, dysphasia, and speech-related events)
- Insomnia

The STAR trial reported that serious adverse events occurred in less than 2% of patients [6]. The most common complaints were related to tongue sensation and stimulation. Eighteen percent of participants had temporary tongue weakness which resolved over a few weeks. Forty percent reported discomfort with stimulation, and 21% reported tongue soreness or abrasions related to stimulation. These symptoms improved in most patients with adjustment of device settings.

7.5 Outcomes

The STAR trial, the initial multicenter trial of 126 patients, showed an average AHI reduction from 32.0 to 15.3 [6]. The ADHERE registry, a large multicenter retrospective and prospective trial that was a follow-up to the STAR trial, enrolled 301 patients and found an average AHI reduction of 35.6–10.2 [12]. Self-reported outcomes included a decrease in Epworth Sleepiness Scale (ESS) and improvement in Functional Outcomes of Sleep Questionnaire (FOSQ). Subsequent 3 and 5 years' follow-up of patients in the STAR trial showed persistent durable response to therapy [7, 8]. Moreover, studies looking at adherence report average usage of 6.5 h a night [12]. This is in stark contrast to adherence to CPAP where reported average usage is around 3.3–3.5 h a night [13, 14].

7.6 Future Directions and Summary

Upper airway stimulation has been shown to be a safe and effective therapy for the treatment of OSA. Its approach has given us new insight into the physiology of OSA and its treatment. Future directions of therapy will likely be directed by better understanding of the neuromuscular physiology in treatment of OSA whether through surgical neurostimulation or other methods.

References

1. Fujita S, Conway W, Zorick F, Roth T. Surgical correction of anatomic azbnormalities in obstructive sleep apnea syndrome: uvulopalatopharyngoplasty. Otolaryngol Head Neck Surg. 1981;89:923–34. https://doi.org/10.1177/019459988108900609.
2. Handler E, Hamans E, Goldberg AN, Mickelson S. Tongue suspension: an evidence-based review and comparison to hypopharyngeal surgery for OSA. Laryngoscope. 2014;124:329–36. https://doi.org/10.1002/lary.24187.
3. Miller SC, Nguyen SA, Ong AA, Gillespie MB. Transoral robotic base of tongue reduction for obstructive sleep apnea: a systematic review and meta-analysis. Laryngoscope. 2017;127:258–65. https://doi.org/10.1002/lary.26060.
4. Stuck BA, Ravesloot MJL, Eschenhagen T, de Vet HCW, Sommer JU. Uvulopalatopharyngoplasty with or without tonsillectomy in the treatment of adult obstructive sleep apnea—a systematic review. Sleep Med. 2018;50:152–65. https://doi.org/10.1016/j.sleep.2018.05.004.
5. Remmers JE, Issa FG, Suratt PM. Sleep and respiration. J Appl Physiol. 1990;68:1286–9. https://doi.org/10.1152/jappl.1990.68.3.1286.
6. Strollo PJ Jr, et al. Upper-airway stimulation for obstructive sleep apnea. N Engl J Med. 2014;370:139–49. https://doi.org/10.1056/NEJMoa1308659.
7. Woodson BT, et al. Three-year outcomes of cranial nerve stimulation for obstructive sleep apnea: the STAR trial. Otolaryngol Head Neck Surg. 2016;154:181–8. https://doi.org/10.1177/0194599815616618.
8. Woodson BT, et al. Upper airway stimulation for obstructive sleep apnea: 5-year outcomes. Otolaryngol Head Neck Surg. 2018;159:194–202. https://doi.org/10.1177/0194599818762383.
9. Friedman M, et al. Targeted hypoglossal nerve stimulation for the treatment of obstructive sleep apnea: six-month results. Laryngoscope. 2016;126:2618–23. https://doi.org/10.1002/lary.25909.
10. Huntley C, et al. Upper airway stimulation in patients with obstructive sleep apnea and an elevated body mass index: a multi-institutional review. Laryngoscope. 2018;128(10):2425–8. https://doi.org/10.1002/lary.27426.
11. Croft CB, Pringle M. Sleep nasendoscopy: a technique of assessment in snoring and obstructive sleep apnoea. Clin Otolaryngol Allied Sci. 1991;16:504–9.
12. Boon M, et al. Upper airway stimulation for obstructive sleep apnea: results from the ADHERE registry. Otolaryngol Head Neck Surg. 2018;159:379–85. https://doi.org/10.1177/0194599818764896.
13. Gottlieb DJ, et al. CPAP versus oxygen in obstructive sleep apnea. N Engl J Med. 2014;370:2276–85. https://doi.org/10.1056/NEJMoa1306766.
14. McEvoy RD, et al. CPAP for prevention of cardiovascular events in obstructive sleep apnea. N Engl J Med. 2016;375:919–31. https://doi.org/10.1056/NEJMoa1606599.

8 Genioglossus Advancement

Reju Joy and Sharon Aronovich

8.1 Introduction

Since the initial description of a mandibular osteotomy procedure to increase the hypopharyngeal space in 1984, genioglossus advancement surgery (GGA) has been used on its own or more commonly in combination with uvulopalatopharyngoplasty (UPPP), hyoid myotomy, and suspension in patients with obstructive sleep apnea (OSA) [1]. In some severe cases of OSA, this procedure is also used in combination with maxillomandibular advancement (MMA). The genioglossus muscle acts as a major pharyngeal dilator and is believed to play a significant role in closure of the airway during sleep-induced hypotonia of oropharyngeal muscles [2]. This muscle plays an important role in retaining an open-air passage in the oropharynx and during sleep; genioglossus activation is influenced by numerous variables, including sleep-wake status, intrapharyngeal negative pressure, blood gases, arousal, respiratory control, and fatigue [3–5].

Fujita used a classification system to describe the level of collapse seen in patients with OSA [6]. Type I describes abnormalities of the upper oropharyngeal airway, including the palate, uvula, and tonsils. Type II consist of upper oropharyngeal and hypopharyngeal airway pathology, and type III involves only the hypopharyngeal airway (i.e., lingual tonsils, tongue base, supraglottis, and hypopharynx). The relevance of targeting the appropriate level of airway collapse was further illustrated by Sher and colleagues, who reported only 5% success in patients with retrolingual (types II and III) collapse who undergo a uvulopalatopharyngoplasty (UPPP) alone [7].

R. Joy
Department of Oral and Maxillofacial Surgery, University of Maryland, Baltimore, MD, USA
e-mail: rjoy@med.umich.edu

S. Aronovich (✉)
Department of Oral and Maxillofacial Surgery, University of Michigan, Ann Arbor, MI, USA
e-mail: saronovi@med.umich.edu

S. O. Salman (ed.), *Modern Management of Obstructive Sleep Apnea*,
https://doi.org/10.1007/978-3-030-11443-5_8

The rationale of GGA surgery is to stabilize the hypopharyngeal airway by the forward movement of the genial tubercle and hence the genioglossus muscle, which will advance the tongue and induce tension at the base of the tongue. This will, therefore, reduce the likelihood of collapse of the tongue backward into the posterior airway during sleep making this a more appropriate procedure for those patients with type II and type III obstruction. In this chapter we will review the relevant anatomy, history of the procedure, its role in current day practice, and different techniques.

8.2 Anatomy

The genioglossus muscle has been extensively scrutinized in the context of obstructive sleep apnea. This is because of its involvement in hypopharyngeal airway collapse and resultant obstructions noted especially during sleep stages with decreased neuromuscular tone (i.e., REM atonia). The genioglossus muscle is a paired, fan-shaped extrinsic tongue muscle. It arises from the superior genial tubercles of the mandible, and occasionally some fibers also take origin from the adjacent surface of the mandible lateral to the superior genial tubercles. The muscle inserts into the body of the hyoid bone, the tip of the tongue and throughout the dorsum of the tongue. The superior fibers retract the tip of the tongue, whereas the middle fibers depress the dorsum of the tongue [8]. The inferior fibers advance the hyoid anterior-superiorly. The muscle is innervated by cranial nerve 12 and receives its major vascular supply from the lingual arteries bilaterally.

The geniohyoid muscle is found just inferior to the genioglossus muscle taking its origin from the inferior genial tubercles. It then runs posteriorly and inferiorly, to be inserted into the anterior surface of the body of the hyoid bone. This muscle also dilates the upper airway through its action of moving the hyoid bone upward and forward.

The genial tubercles are bony spines on the lingual surface of the mandible near the midline, and there are two pairs. The superior genial spines are almost always paired bilaterally although on occasions they are found fused together. In contrast, the right and left inferior genial spines were usually indistinguishable. The anatomy of the genial tubercles, especially its relation to the apices of the lower central incisors is of utmost importance in the context of GGA surgery. Although radiographs may give an indication of the relation of the mandibular incisors to the genial tubercles, there is an approximate magnification of 8% in periapical radiographs and 30% in panoramic radiographs. Therefore, preoperative assessment with three-dimensional imaging is preferred.

A cadaver study by Silverstein and Costello found the average distance from the apex of the incisors to the genial tubercle was 11.8 mm with a range of 9–15 mm [8]. However, another anatomical assessment using measurements from CT scans and dry cadaveric skulls found the average distance between the apices of the roots of the mandibular central incisors to the superior genial tubercles was 6.45 mm [9]. The same study also observed that 35% of the genial tubercles were situated within 5 mm from the apices of the mandibular incisor teeth which may increase the risk for devitalization of teeth as determined by Bell's angiographic studies [10]. In

1988, morphological measurements on ten human cadaver half-heads found a range of 2.5–13 mm (mean 6.83 mm) between the incisor apex and the superior genioglossus muscle attachment [11]. Our clinical experience is consistent with a wide variation in genial tubercle positions and tooth root lengths that require identification with three-dimensional (3D) imaging.

8.3 History and Evolution of the GGA Technique

The first procedure described by Riley et al. in 1984 employed an intraoral approach, and the osteotomy design was similar to an advancement genioplasty [1]. The hyoid bone was also fixed to the inferior border of the mandible after myotomy of the infrahyoid muscles. This is referred to as the genioglossus advancement/hyoid myotomy. This procedure was further modified by Riley and colleagues in 1986 to retain the continuity of the lower border of the mandible by limiting the osteotomy to a rectangular window of the bone in the anterior mandible containing the genial tubercles and genioglossus muscle complex [12]. The bone-muscle flap is advanced and rotated 30–45° to create bone overlap for a fixation screw (Fig. 8.1). This was referred to as the anterior mandibular osteotomy. This modification reduced the risk of fracture of the mandible which was reported in prior techniques. However, rotation of the flap may create excessive tension possibly resulting in detachment of the muscle complex. One of the other limitations of this procedure is the risk of injury or devitalization of the anterior mandibular dentition.

Variations of this procedure include different types of osteotomies and alteration in transposition of the bone segment [12–18]. In 1993 Riley et al. put forward the Stanford protocol where each patient was classified according to the site of obstruction (type I, oropharynx; type II, oropharynx/hypopharynx; and type III, hypopharynx) [13]. In phase I surgery, patients with type I obstruction (soft palate) receive UPPP, and patients with type III obstruction (base of tongue) receive genioglossus advancement/hyoid myotomy (GAHM). Patients with type II (palate and base of tongue) receive UPPP and GAHM together. Patients who failed phase I surgical

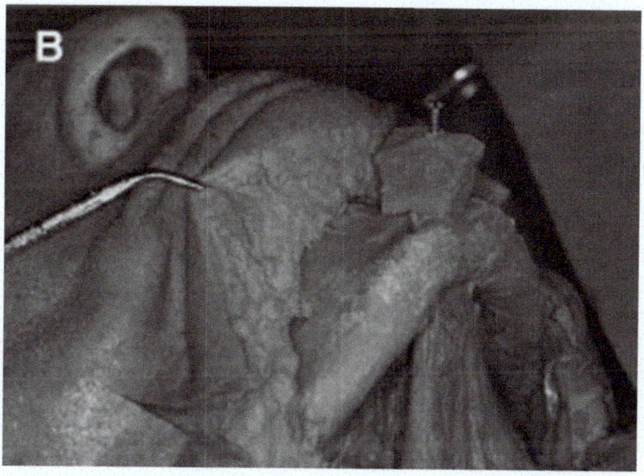

Fig. 8.1 Cadaver dissection demonstrating a rectangular osteotomy with genioglossus muscle placed under tension via advancement and rotation (Reprinted with permission from Li KK, Riley RW, Powell NB et al. Obstructive sleep apnea surgery: Genioglossus advancement revisited. *J Oral Maxillofac Surg*. 2001; 59:1181–1184)

procedures were then recruited into phase II where they were offered maxillomandibular advancement (MMA) surgery.

In 1998, David Dattilo designed the mandibular trapezoid osteotomy through an extraoral approach to allow the maximum advancement of the musculature in a natural and functional position while minimizing esthetic profile changes to the lower facial third [14].

In 2000, Lee and Woodson introduced the Genial Bone Advancement Trephine (GBAT) system (Stryker Leibinger Corporation) which boasted greater ease of isolation and advancement of the genioglossus muscle [15]. This system incorporated a guide plate and trephine (12–14 mm) to create a circular osteotomy for capture of the genial tubercles. A prebent fixation plate matches the osteotomized segment, allowing for advancement and fixation with minimal manipulation. The proponents of this technique claim reduced operating time, fewer postoperative complications, and reliable capture of the genial tubercles. However, localization of the tubercles was based on panoramic radiographs and palpation only.

In 2001, Hendler et al. proposed the mortised genioplasty technique with the goal of achieving greater expansion of the hypopharyngeal airway through advancement of the genioglossus, geniohyoid, mylohyoid, and anterior belly of digastric muscles simultaneously (Fig. 8.2). This technique uses a rectangular box superiorly to capture the genial tubercles, with the inferior aspect of the box extended laterally as in a standard genioplasty technique. Fixation is applied laterally on both sides to lessen the risk of mandibular fracture [16]. This technique is ideally suited for patients who benefit esthetically from a genioplasty advancement. Despite the hypothesized airway expansion described by the authors, changes in airway dimensions have not been studied. Moreover, compared to a window technique which is limited to capturing the genial tubercle attachments, the mortised genioplasty may be more susceptible to relapse given a stronger posterior muscle pull and bony

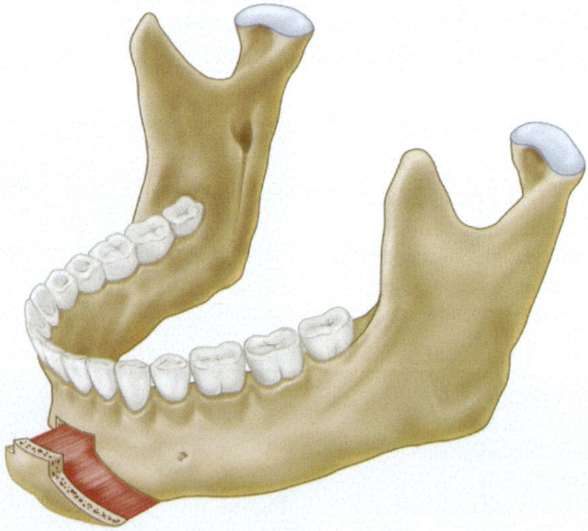

Fig. 8.2 Mortised genioglossus advancement design to capture the genioglossus, geniohyoid, and anterior digastric muscles (Reprinted with permission from Silverstein K, Costello BJ, Giannakkpoulos H, et al. Genioglossus muscle attachments: An anatomic analysis and the implications for genioglossus advancement. *Oral Surg Oral Med Oral Pathol Oral Radiol Endod.* 90: 687, 2000)

union limited to the superior border of the osteotomy. Interestingly, relapse of anterior segmental osteotomies for GGA have not been studied.

In 2009, Demian and colleagues described a technique that allows complete capture and advancement of the genial tubercles along with the entire genioglossus complex without noticeable changes in the soft tissue esthetics [17]. This is accomplished by carrying the horizontal osteotomy to just medial of the canine roots and extending the vertical cuts to the inferior border. The whole complex is advanced and the buccal cortex and cancellous bone removed, leaving the lingual cortex with the attached musculature. This is then fixed with a prebent plate across the inferior border to minimize alteration in chin contour. The authors claim this technique combines the advantages of inferior mandibular osteotomy procedure and the rectangular box osteotomy.

Another modification of the conventional rectangular GGA osteotomy describes the creation of a bony groove in the basal bone inferior to the osteotomy in order to accommodate the muscle complex while maximizing the advancement with fixation of the lingual plate using positional screws anterior and inferior (to the window osteotomy) over the inferior border [18]. This technique avoids the 90° rotation which places torquing stress on the muscle attachment at the tubercle and increases the risk of detachment or vascular compromise. For patients with mild retrogenia, the authors also claim a more pleasing aesthetic outcome as compared to the latter technique which may blunt the labiomental fold [18].

8.4 Preoperative Evaluation

Patients considered for surgical treatment of OSA undergo a complete medical history and physical examination, fill out validated instruments to assess hypersomnolence (Epworth Sleepiness Scale) and sleep quality (Pittsburgh sleep quality index), undergo a polysomnogram (PSG) to establish the diagnosis and severity of sleep-disordered breathing, and have an assessment of the upper airway via fiberoptic nasoendoscopy and cone beam computed tomography (CBCT).

Exam findings which increase the risk of OSA include obesity, adenotonsillary hypertrophy, retrognathia, micrognathia, macroglossia, a low hyoid position, elongated soft palate, deviation of the nasal septum, turbinate hypertrophy, a thick short neck, or mass lesions in the nasopharynx or hypopharynx. Conditions like trisomy 21, myxedema, goiter, acromegaly, and lymphoma may be associated with OSA, owing to their effects on the upper airway anatomy.

PSG: A full-night polysomnography is carried out to assess the following parameters—total sleep time, sleep stages NREM and REM (via electrooculogram), as well as percent of sleep in each, electroencephalography, chest and abdominal movements, snoring, nasal airflow, lowest oxygen saturation, lower limb movement (via electromyography), and electrocardiographic activity. The severity as an index is summarized as apnea-hypopnea index (AHI).

Fiberoptic nasoendoscopy is performed to determine the extent of airway obstruction while the patient is supine at rest and during forced inspiration or

Mueller maneuver. Posterior septal deviation, enlargement of the inferior turbinate, and nasopharyngeal lesions are some of the abnormalities that may be better appreciated by endoscopic evaluation. The Mueller maneuver is performed while the patient is upright with a closed mouth and pinched nose with maximum inspiration. The increased intraluminal negative pressure with this maneuver attempts to duplicate the sleep-related pressure changes to more accurately assess the presence of dynamic upper airway collapse. Because the patient is awake when this is performed, and upper airway muscles maintain their tone, false-positive and false-negative results are possible [19]. A five-point scale provides a more objective measure to rate the sites of collapse during the Mueller maneuver to increase its reliability [20].

CBCT: Visualization of the upper airway with CBCT scans provides important 3-dimensional information about surrounding structures and their contribution to, as well as the specific location of, airway obstruction [21]. Airway space measurements, including volume and cross-sectional area, have been shown to be quite accurate by use of CBCT scans. Multivariate analysis shows both retroglossal space and retropalatal space narrowing to be predictive of an elevated respiratory disturbance Index (RDI) [22]. The relationship between the airway area and the likelihood of OSA has been previously demonstrated [23]. Finally a CBCT is used for virtual surgical planning including intraoperative osteotomy design and positioning or cutting guides which allows precise capture of the genial tubercle, while avoiding injury to key surrounding structures [24].

Hueman et al. in their effort to determine the accuracy of CBCT to predict the location of the genial tubercle looked into the width of the genial tubercle, genial tubercle height, distance from inferior border of mandible to genial tubercle, mandibular height, and mandibular thickness. No significant difference was found in mean distances between cadaver dissections vs the 3D cone beam CT [25].

8.5 Virtual Surgical Planning

There have been various attempts to study the anatomy of the genial tubercles to design the perfect osteotomy that would incorporate maximum capture of the tubercles along with the muscle complex while minimizing the risks of instrumenting in proximity to the apices of adjacent mandibular teeth. Given the anatomical variability between individuals, the ideal osteotomy design should be customized to suit the individual situation.

Over the past few years, the use of virtual surgical planning (VSP) and computer-aided design and manufacturing (CAD/CAM) has created a paradigm shift in the diagnosis and planning of orthognathic and craniofacial procedures. The authors now regularly employ virtual surgical planning in all GGA procedures to enable 3-dimensional visualization in order to confirm the feasibility of the procedure. For this purpose, DICOM files containing CBCT data and stone models or STL files of an intraoral scan are obtained. Patient with an excessively thin symphysis <8 mm (A-P dimension) or those with <5 mm of vertical clearance between the superior

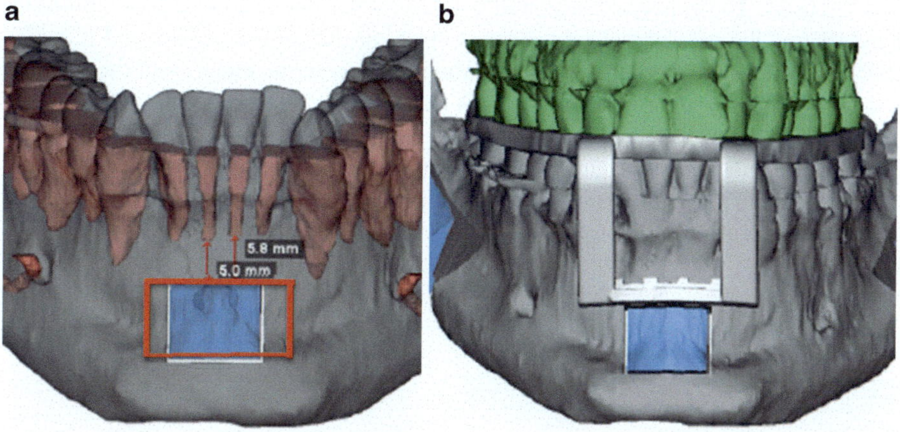

Fig. 8.3 (**a**) Example of a case where the superior aspect of the genial tubercle is 5 mm away from the lower incisor root apex. Further lateral extension (red outline) from the marked osteotomy lines enables greater muscle capture and facilitates bony overlap when rotating the rectangular window. (**b**) Example of a cutting guide to place the osteotomy just above the genial tubercles while clearing the mandibular incisor apices

genial tubercles and the incisor root apices are not considered good candidates for GGA. Preoperative planning includes osteotomy design and fabrication of cutting guides via rapid prototyping technology to ensure complete capture of the genioglossus muscle while decreasing the risk of neurosensory alterations, dental injury, and mandibular fracture (Fig. 8.3a, b).

8.6 Surgical Technique

Genioglossus advancement (GGA) is typically performed transorally. The mandibular anterior vestibule is injected with a local anesthetic containing epinephrine for hemostasis and to prevent surgical sensitization. With anterior traction on the lower lip, a mucosal incision is made approximately 10 mm below the mucogingival junction in the gingivolabial sulcus. This is carried out with a gentle smiling curve and extended to the distal aspect of the canine teeth. The incisions carried through mucosa, submucosa, and mentalis muscle and periosteum. An adequate cuff of mentalis muscle is left attached to proximal periosteum to facilitate soft tissue closure. Dissection is performed subperiosteally to expose the mandibular symphysis. Lateral dissection to expose the mental nerves is not required unless the osteotomy is carried to the inferior border posteriorly. [1, 14, 16, 17]

Prior to osteotomy, the mandible may be stabilized to the maxillary arch with maxillomandibular fixation (MMF) wires. If a cutting guide is used, this is inserted first and stabilized with MMF wires. The chosen osteotomy design is then performed with a sagittal saw and/or a reciprocating saw as needed under copious irrigation. Alternatively, a piezoelectric or ultrasonic handpiece with a straight blade may be used. The superior horizontal osteotomy should ideally be a minimum of 5 mm below the mandibular root apices to prevent incisor root injury, and if applicable, the inferior horizontal osteotomy should preserve the integrity of the inferior border to minimize the risk of fractures. A custom cutting guide based on the virtual plan is essential to predictably capture the genioglossus muscle and avoid damage to adjacent teeth. Since the canine roots are significantly more elongated relative to the incisors, the vertical bone cuts are made just medial to the canine tooth to avoid root injury. Before completing the osteotomy, a titanium screw is placed in the outer cortex to control and manipulate the bone flap (Fig. 8.4a–e). The full-thickness osteotomy should be completed with the sagittal saw instead of osteotomes and mallets

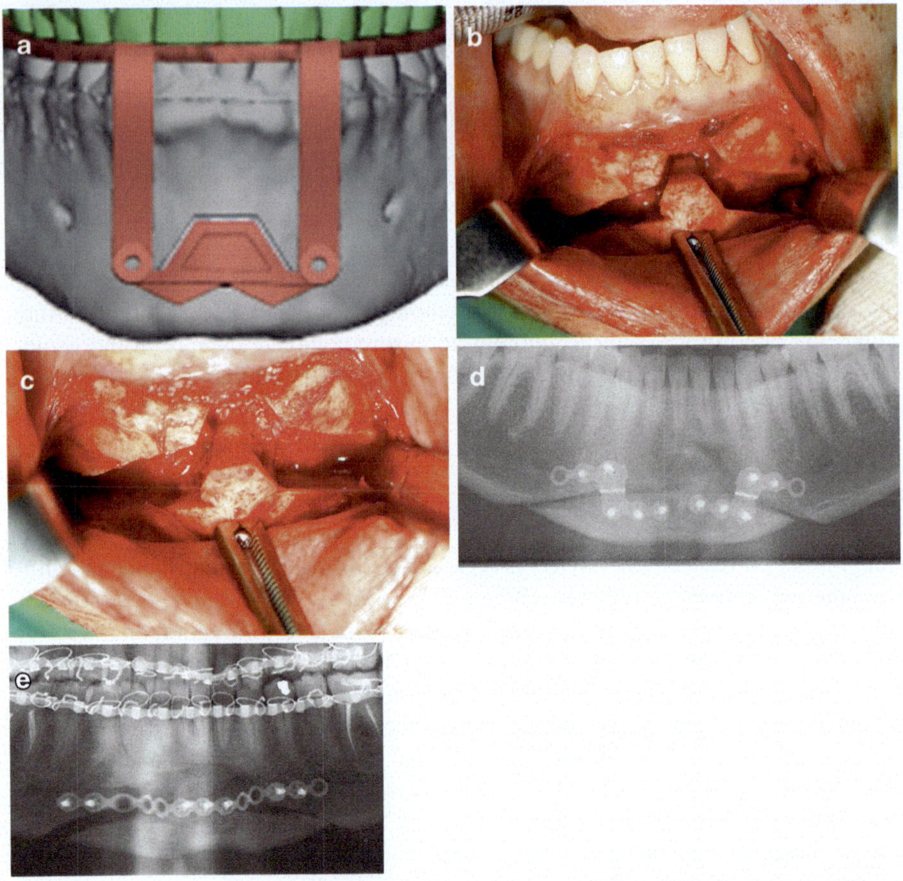

Fig. 8.4 (**a**) Virtually planned cutting guide allows precise placement of the superior osteotomy. (**b**) This case demonstrates a mortised genioplasty that includes lateral extensions to the inferior border as in a standard genioplasty. (**c**) Closer inspection reveals the genioglossus muscle attachment at the genial tubercle near the superior edge of the osteotomy. (**d**) Fixation may be achieved with two lateral plates and screws. (**e**) Alternative fixation method with a straight chain plate bent to adapt to the surrounding bones and overlying soft tissues

to avoid premature separation of the buccal cortex and marrow from the lingual cortex. In the window technique, the vertical and horizontal osteotomies should be parallel to each other. The osteotomized bony segment is delivered anteriorly by gentle traction until the lingual cortex including the insertion of genioglossus muscle reaches the anterior aspect of the mandible. The lingual aspect is inspected to confirm that the genioglossus muscle was captured in the bone flap.

The mandibular outer cortex and marrow of the repositioned segment are then removed using a reciprocating saw, while the lingual plate is stabilized with a bone-holding forceps. The osteotomized segment is then secured anteriorly using one of the methods described above.

After good hemostasis has been achieved, the surgical site is closed in two layers with the mentalis muscle resuspended with slowly absorbable sutures, and the mucosal edges are approximated with interrupted absorbable sutures on a tapered needle. A mentalis support dressing is adapted with elastic tape bandage, and light pressure is applied with a head wrap. This is used to prevent postoperative hematoma and lower lip or chin ptosis. The patient should be placed on a pureed to soft diet during the healing period.

8.7 Perioperative Complications

Depending on the technique adopted for GGA, several complications have been reported. These include mandibular fractures, injury and devitalization of adjacent mandibular teeth, neurosensory disturbances in the mental nerve distribution including dysesthesia, floor of mouth hematoma, infection, exposed hardware, unfavorable or unesthetic facial changes including lip ptosis, detachment of genioglossus muscle from the lingual plate, lack of improvement or worsening sleep parameters (AHI, minimum oxygen saturation, etc.), and lack of improvement in sleep quality and/or sleep-related symptoms.

8.8 Outcomes

One of the earliest studies employing GGA as a procedure to treat OSA was a review of 55 patients with OSA who were treated with GGA and hyoid myotomy with suspension (GAHM) [26]. They observed a response rate of 67% based on a mean reduction in RDI from 58.7 ± 23.4 to 11.8 ± 6.9. Since the introduction of GGA by Riley, the technique has undergone many modifications over the last 30 years to improve outcomes and limit complications [12–18]. However, the combination of GGA with other hypopharyngeal or oropharyngeal procedures is often necessary to adequately treat OSA, making direct comparisons between isolated procedures difficult. The majority of outcome studies on the effectiveness of GGA for the treatment of OSA have been limited to case series and retrospective studies (level four evidence). A review of literature shows success in the range between 40 and 70% where success is determined as postoperative respiratory disturbance index (RDI) less than 20 with at least a 50% reduction relative to the preoperative polysomnogram (known as Sher's success criteria) [7, 27–30].

Thus far, two systematic reviews have carried out a meta-analysis for outcomes of hypopharyngeal procedures in patients with OSA. In 2006, a meta-analysis by Kezirian and Goldberg [31] found success rates of genioglossal advancement to be between 39% and 78% after evaluating four case series totaling 91 cases [32–35]. Results of GGA as a sole procedure for treatment of hypopharyngeal obstruction in patients with severe OSA revealed a success rate of more than 60% in three studies [33–35]. Only two studies investigated lowest oxyhemoglobin saturation results [33, 35], and both showed improvement in low oxyhemoglobin saturation (LSAT). While there is evidence of improved outcomes with surgery, careful patient selection can significantly affect the success of treatment.

The second of the two systematic reviews evaluated the outcomes of various GGA techniques combined with hyoid surgery as treatment for OSA. Patients with hypoventilation syndrome or central sleep apnea and patients who lost more than 10% of their body weight between polysomnograms were excluded. Sher's surgical success criteria were used, and a surgical cure was defined as a postoperative AHI < 5 events/h. They identified 4 studies (45 patients) in which genioplasty was performed [36–39], 5 studies (24 patients) in which GTA was performed [18, 30, 32, 33, 40], and 4 studies (50 patients) in which genial tubercle advancement (GTA) with hyoid surgery was performed [1, 12, 26, 41]. A meta-analysis revealed four main findings. First, a comparison of the mean AHI before and after surgery demonstrated a reduction of 41.7% in patients with isolated GGA, 48.6% in patients who had genioplasty, and 57.4% in patients who underwent GGA with hyoid surgery. Second, LSAT scores in all studies showed an increase after surgery regardless of technique. Third, GTA demonstrated a greater improvement in AHI and LSAT following the procedure when compared to a genioplasty. The authors attributed a higher variability with genioplasty outcomes due to various modifications of technique allowing for different percentage of capture of the genial tubercles. The authors hypothesized that any technique that allows for complete capture of the genial tubercles and avoids excessive subperiosteal dissection of the inferior symphysis could result in similar outcomes to that of GTA. Fourth, although both GGA and genioplasty potentially increase the size of the upper airway by anteriorly displacing the tongue, the addition of hyoid surgery addresses another dimension of the obstruction, which is the reduction of the length of the upper airway. This lends further support to multilevel surgery compared to isolated procedures in OSA patients.

Hendler et al. achieved a success of 48% in their series of 33 patients who underwent the mortised genioplasty [16]. They observed patients with a BMI < 30 had a more successful outcome compared to patients with BMI > 30. Similarly, patients with preoperative AHI less than 50 had a more successful outcome (71%) compared to patients with a preoperative AHI greater than 50 (32%).

Kuscu and colleagues studied isolated GGA results for patients with a retrospective analysis and noted a 53% success rate based on AHI [30]. The authors also noted an improvement in ESS score and no significant difference between pre- and postoperative values of BMI and minimum O_2 saturation.

There is evidence that GGA may reduce hypersomnolence. A prospective randomized study by Thomas and colleagues comparing GGA with tongue-base suspension demonstrated a reduction in Epworth Sleepiness Scale (ESS) scores in the GGA group (eight patients) from a mean of 13.3 to 5.4. Airway collapse for five of eight patients measured on Muller maneuver improved by a mean of 75% at the base of the tongue [42].

Finally, while several studies have evaluated the effects of maxillomandibular advancement on the upper airway with 2D and 3D imaging, the influence of GGA on the airway remains poorly understood. In one Brazilian study of ten nonobese patients with mild to moderate OSA, baseline and postoperative posterior airway space (PAS) measurements were carried out on lateral cephalometric radiographs after GGA. A statistically significant increase in PAS from 7.9 ± 2.3 mm and 10.8 ± 2.5 mm was noted ($p < 0.001$). Moreover, this correlated with a reduction in AHI from 12.4 ± 4.6 to 4.4 ± 5.7 ($p < 0.001$) and a success rate of 70% [43]. While patients with airway narrowing seem to be good candidates for surgery, Johnson et al. noted that a narrower airway was associated with a smaller change in AHI, while patients with larger PAS had greater changes in AHI. They concluded that a smaller PAS was associated with treatment failure; however, their study was limited by a small sample size, a wide range of preoperative AHI, and an obese population [33]. Importantly, they were not able to identify any other predictive variables that correlated with change in AHI. In a critical assessment of responders and non-responders to GAHS, Riley and colleagues noted that non-responders ($n = 18$) had a higher incidence of chronic obstructive lung disease and greater mandibular retrognathia with a mean SNB angle of 75.5 ± 1.5 compared to the responder group (mean SNB 81 ± 2.0). Although they did not clarify what statistical methodology was used to determine the predictive value of COPD and SNB, they concluded that patients with normal skeletal development were better candidates for GAHS [26]. Implicit in this observation is the possible need for mandibular advancement in the presence of significant mandibular retrognathia.

Given the variability in response to surgery, a predictive tool akin to a CPAP titration would be quite beneficial. In one attempt to identify a predictive tool, Barrera et al. investigated the role of intraoperative bone flap tension and bicortical width of the mandible on surgical success of GGA. The authors measured the bicortical width of mandible at the genial tubercles intraoperatively and the force required to pull the osteotomized bony window forward with a tensiometer. Out of 18 patients, the authors found a 61.1% success rate. The variables of tension and bicortical width independently had no impact on postoperative outcomes. However, they noted a lower tension to width ratio was significantly associated with surgical response in their patients. Unfortunately, since the tension is determined intraoperatively, it cannot serve a predictive role in the preoperative setting [44].

8.9 Summary of Recommendations

Based on the available polysomnographic and surgical data, the following are general guidelines for the use of GGA surgery

1. A significant number of patients with severe OSA continue to have moderate to severe OSA (AHI >15) after GGA surgery. Patients with mild to moderate OSA have the highest success rate with GGA. MMA should be considered for patients with severe OSA.
2. Younger patients (<35) may have better airway soft tissue response and might experience higher success compared to older patients.
3. Patients with lower body weight, BMI <30, have better results with GGA.
4. The role of tongue size remains controversial. One study indicates that relative macroglossia predicts surgical success; however excess macroglossia or glossoptosis may predict poor outcomes with GGA.
5. Patients with microgenia may see a benefit in facial esthetics depending on the technique employed.
6. Patients with severe retrognathia (SNA <72) and significant upper airway narrowing may not respond to GGA but may be considered for MMA.
7. Due to substantial variability in the position of the genial tubercles, use of anatomical averages for GGA osteotomies may fail to capture the whole muscle attachment and increases the risk of damage to adjacent dentition. The use of virtual surgical planning can help determine suitable candidates for the procedure and allow for accurate capture of the tubercles and muscle complex.

8.10 Summary

Genioglossus advancement is a technique-sensitive procedure that requires a tailored approach using virtual surgical planning and 3D printed cutting guides to identify an isolated tubercle instead of relying on averages. The authors feel genioglossus advancement has a role as an adjunctive procedure in conjunction with MMA, as well as other retropharyngeal and retropalatal procedures. However, both as an adjunctive procedure and on its own, its true value in long-term and short-term reduction of AHI and improvement of sleep parameters is yet to be fully determined.

Based on the evidence so far, an ideal patient for GGA would be a young patient who is not obese, has mild to moderate OSA, and does not have significant airway compromise related to macroglossia, retrognathia, or neuromuscular tone involvement.

References

1. Riley R, Guilleminault C, Powell N, Derman S. Mandibular osteotomy and hyoid bone advancement for obstructive sleep apnea: a case report. Sleep. 1984;7:79–82.
2. Sauerland EK, Harper RM. The human tongue during sleep: electromyographic activity of the genioglossus muscle. Exp Neurol. 1976;51:160–70.
3. Lo YL, Jordan AS, Malhotra A, et al. Genioglossal muscle response to CO_2 stimulation during NREM sleep. Sleep. 2006;29:470–7.
4. Bianchi AL, Denavit Saubie M, Champagnat J. Central control of breathing in mammals: neuronal circuitry, membrane properties, and neurotransmitters. Physiol Rev. 1995;75:1–45.

5. Stanchina ML, Malhotra A, Fogel RB, et al. The influence of lung volume on pharyngeal mechanics, collapsibility, and genioglossus muscle activation during sleep. Sleep. 2003;26:851–6.
6. Fujita S. Pharyngeal surgery for obstructive sleep apnea and snoring. In: Fairbanks DNF, et al., editors. Snoring and obstructive sleep apnea. New York: Raven Press; 1987. p. 101–28.
7. Sher AE, Schechtman KB, Piccirillo JF. The efficacy of surgical modifications of the upper airway in adults with obstructive sleep apnea syndrome. Sleep. 1996;19(2):156–77.
8. Silverstein K, Costello BJ, Giannakpoulos H, Hendler B. Genioglossus muscle attachments: an anatomic analysis and the implications for genioglossus advancement. Oral Surg Oral Med Oral Pathol Oral Radiol Endod. 2000;90:686–8.
9. Mintz SM, Ettinger AC, Geist JR, Geist RY. Anatomic relationship of the genial tubercles to the dentition as determined by cross-sectional tomography. J Oral Maxillofac Surg. 1995;53:1324–6.
10. Bell WH, Proffit WR, White RP. Surgical correction of dentofacial deformities. 1st ed. Philadelphia, PA: Saunders; 1980. p. 1218–26.
11. Zhang X, Bell WH, Washko PW. Relationship of mandibular anterior tooth apices to genial muscle attachments. Oral Surg Oral Med Oral Pathol. 1988;65:653.
12. Riley R, Powell N, Guilleminault C. Inferior sagittal osteotomy of the mandible with hyoid myotomy-suspension: a new procedure for obstructive sleep apnea. Otolaryngol Head Neck Surg. 1986;94:589–93.
13. Riley RW, Powell NB, Guilleminault C. Obstructive sleep apnea syndrome: a review of 306 consecutively treated surgical patients. Otolaryngol Head Neck Surg. 1993;108:117–25.
14. Dattilo DJ. The mandibular trapezoid osteotomy for the treatment of obstructive sleep apnea: report of a case. J Oral Maxillofac Surg. 1998;56:1442–6.
15. Lee NR, Woodson BT. Genioglossus muscle advancement via a trephine osteotomy approach. Oper Tech Otolaryngol Head Neck Surg. 2000;11(50):50–4.
16. Hendler BH, Costello BJ, Silverstein K, et al. A protocol for uvulopalatopharyngoplasty, mortised genioplasty, and maxillomandibular advancement in patients with obstructive sleep apnea: an analysis of 40 cases. J Oral Maxillofac Surg. 2001;59:892–7.
17. Demian NM, Alford J, Takashima M. An alternative technique for genioglossus muscle advancement in phase I surgery in the treatment of obstructive sleep apnea. J Oral Maxillofac Surg. 2009;67(10):2315–8.
18. Garcia Vega JR, de la Plata MM, Galindo N, et al. Genioglossus muscle advancement: a modification of the conventional technique. J Craniomaxillofac Surg. 2014;42(3):239–44.
19. Hsu PP, Tan BY, Chan YH, et al. Clinical predictors in obstructive sleep apnea patients with computer assisted quantitative video endoscopic upper airway analysis. Laryngoscope. 2004;114:791–9.
20. Terris DJ, Hanasono MM, Liu YC. Reliability of the Muller maneuver and its association with sleep disordered breathing. Laryngoscope. 2000;110:1819–23.
21. Schendel S. The airway assessment of the patient with obstructive sleep apnea. In: Surgical enhancement of orthodontic treatment, vol. 47. Craniofacial Growth Series. Ann Arbor, MI: University of Michigan; 2009. p. 203–30.
22. Yamashina A, Tanimoto K, Sutthiprapaporn P. The reliability of computed tomography (CT) values and dimensional measurements of the oropharyngeal region using cone beam CT comparison with multivector CT. Dent Maxillofac Radiol. 2008;37:245.
23. Li HY, Chen NH, Wang CR, Shu YH, Wang PC. Use of three-dimensional computed tomography scan to evaluate upper airway patency for patients undergoing sleep-disordered breathing surgery. Otolaryngol Head Neck Surg. 2003;129(4):336–42.
24. Liu SY-C, Huon L-K, Zaghi S, Riley R, Torre C. An accurate method of designing and performing individual-specific genioglossus advancement. Otolaryngol Head Neck Surg. 2017;156(1):194–7.
25. Hueman EM, Noujeim ME, Langlais RP, Prihoda TJ, Miller FR. Accuracy of cone beam computed tomography in determining the location of the genial tubercle. Otolaryngol Head Neck Surg. 2007;137(1):115–8.

26. Riley RW, Powell NB, Guilleminault C. Inferior mandibular osteotomy and hyoid myotomy suspension for obstructive sleep apnea: a review of 55 patients. J Oral Maxillofac Surg. 1989;47:159–64.
27. Ramirez SG, Loube DI. Inferior sagittal osteotomy with hyoid bone suspension for obese patients with sleep apnea. Arch Otolaryngol Head Neck Surg. 1996;122(9):953–7.
28. Vilaseca I, Morello A, Montserrat JM, et al. Usefulness of uvulopalatopharyngoplasty with genioglossus and hyoid advancement in the treatment of obstructive sleep apnea. Arch Otolaryngol Head Neck Surg. 2002;128(4):435–40.
29. Riley RW, Powell NB, Guilleminault C. Obstructive sleep apnea syndrome: a surgical protocol for dynamic upper airway reconstruction. J Oral Maxillofac Surg. 1993;51(7):742–7.
30. Kuscu O, Suslu AE, Ozer S, Gunaydin RO, Ogretmenoglu O, Onerc IM. Sole effect of genioglossus advancement on apnea hypopnea index of patients with obstructive sleep apnea. Acta Otolaryngol. 2015;135:835–9.
31. Kezirian EJ, Goldberg AN. Hypopharyngeal surgery in obstructive sleep apnea: an evidence-based medicine review. Arch Otolaryngol Head Neck Surg. 2006;132(2):206–13.
32. Riley RW, Powell NB, Guilleminault C. Obstructive sleep apnea and the hyoid: a revised surgical procedure. Otolaryngol Head Neck Surg. 1994;111:717–21.
33. Johnson NT, Chinn J. Uvulopalatopharyngoplasty and inferior sagittal mandibular osteotomy with genioglossus advancement for treatment of obstructive sleep apnea. Chest. 1994;105:278–83.
34. Lee NR, Givens CD Jr, Wilson J, Robins RB. Staged surgical treatment of obstructive sleep apnea syndrome: a review of 35 patients. J Oral Maxillofac Surg. 1999;57:382–5.
35. Miller FR, Watson D, Boseley M. The role of the Genial Bone Advancement Trephine system in conjunction with uvulopalatopharyngoplasty in the multilevel management of obstructive sleep apnea. Otolaryngol Head Neck Surg. 2004;130:73–9.
36. Krekmanov L, Andersson L, Ringqvist M, et al. Anterior–inferior mandibular osteotomy in treatment of obstructive sleep apnea syndrome. Int J Adult Orthodon Orthognath Surg. 1998;13:289–98.
37. Santos JF Jr, Abrahao M, Gregorio LC, Zonato AI, Gumieiro EH. Genioplasty for genioglossus muscle advancement in patients with obstructive sleep apnea-hypopnea syndrome and mandibular retrognathia. Braz J Otorhinolaryngol. 2007;73:480–6.
38. Tabrizi R, Pourdanesh F, Soleimanpour M, Shafie E. Evaluation of mandibular wing osteotomy in obstructive sleep apnea cases with retrognathia. J Maxillofac Oral Surg. 2015;14:46–50.
39. Yin W, Feng S, Guan W. Mandibular advancement for the treatment of micrognathia with obstructive sleep apnea. Zhonghua Zheng Xing Shao Shang Wai Ke Za Zhi. 1994;10:265–9.
40. Foltan R, Sonka K. [Genioglossal advancement in the surgical treatment of obstructive sleep apnea syndrome in adults]. Sb Lek. 2000; 101:393–8.
41. Foltan R, Hoffmannova J, Pretl M, Donev F, Vlk M. Genioglossus advancement and hyoid myotomy in treating obstructive sleep apnoea syndrome: a follow-up study. J Craniomaxillofac Surg. 2007;35:246–51.
42. Thomas AJ, Chavoya M, Terris DJ. Preliminary findings from a prospective, randomized trial of two tongue-base surgeries for sleep-disordered breathing. Otolaryngol Head Neck Surg. 2003;129(5):539–46.
43. Santos Junior JF, Abrahao M, Gregorio LC, Zonato AL, Gummieiro EH, et al. Genioplasty for genioglossus advancement in patients with obstructive sleep apnea hypopnea syndrome and mandibular retrognathia. Braz J Otorhinolaryngol. 2007;73(4):480–6.
44. Barrera JE, Dion GR. Predicting surgical response using tensiometry in OSA patients after genioglossus advancement with uvulopalatopharyngoplasty. Otolaryngol Head Neck Surg. 2016;154(3):558–63.

9 Maxillomandibular Advancement

Stacey Nedrud and Salam O. Salman

9.1 Introduction

Untreated obstructive sleep apnea (OSA) has extensive severe consequences, as have been well delineated in previous chapters. Moderate to severe OSA can be blamed for excessive daytime somnolence, poor work performance and occupational injury, motor vehicle accidents, decreased subjective quality of life, neurocognitive impairment, cardiovascular complications, and metabolic and respiratory derangements, among other sequelae [1, 2].

Treatment should be approached in conservative echelons. Viable nonsurgical options such as weight loss, changes in sleep posture, oral appliances, pharmacologic therapy, external nasal support devices, and continuous positive airway pressure (CPAP) should be trialed prior to surgical intervention in most cases [3]. The broad spectrum of surgical modalities can also be approached in a stepwise fashion. However depending on severity and clinical presentation, surgical options are not necessarily performed in ascending order [2]. Surgical options are multitudinous and include tracheostomy, uvulopalatopharyngoplasty (UPPP), laser-assisted uvuloplasty (LAUP), internal and external nasal reconstruction, tonsillectomy and adenoidectomy, base of tongue surgery, hyoid suspension and advancement, varying mandibular osteotomies, genioglossus advancement, maxillary and mandibular advancement (MMA), and others [2–4]. The American Academy of Sleep Medicine has established detailed clinical practice parameters for the diagnosis and surgical treatment of OSA that can help guide the surgeon [1, 5–7]. The American Academy of Oral Maxillofacial Surgeons parameters of care guidelines for the treatment of maxillofacial skeletal deformities updated in 2017 delineate maxillary and mandibular advancement as a successful treatment modality for adult OSA [2].

S. Nedrud · S. O. Salman (✉)
Department of Oral and Maxillofacial Surgery, College of Medicine, University of Florida—Jacksonville, Jacksonville, FL, USA
e-mail: stacey.nedrud@jax.ufl.edu; salam.salman@jax.ufl.edu

S. O. Salman (ed.), *Modern Management of Obstructive Sleep Apnea*,
https://doi.org/10.1007/978-3-030-11443-5_9

9.2 History

The surgical treatment for severe obstructive sleep apnea has evolved dramatically in the past 50 years. As recently as the 1970s and 1980s, a permanent tracheostomy was the most common and efficacious treatment modality, bypassing all potential sites of airway obstruction [3]. Now, tracheostomies are rarely performed in this setting due to the risk of tracheal stenosis, trachea-innominate artery fistula hemorrhages, recurrent bronchitis, speech deficits, and aesthetic concerns [3]. In 1981, Fujita et al. published articles describing UPPP as a primary treatment, but this was soon found to have low success rates: improvement was seen in 50% of patients undergoing UPPP, but complete control of symptoms was only seen in 25–30% [8–12]. Dr. William Bell foresaw the utility of orthognathic surgery as a definitive treatment for OSA, predicting maxillary and mandibular advancement was the next paradigm shift [8]. MMA began to develop in the mid-1980s, when mandibular surgery was found to successfully reverse the symptoms of OSA [8, 9]. Since then, the field has been advanced by many contemporaries and has shown great success in the treatment of severe obstructive sleep apnea.

9.3 Relevant Surgical Anatomy

The relevant airway anatomy in the evaluation for surgical management of obstructive sleep apnea can largely be simplified into three broad categories: nasal, retropalatal, and retroglossal [13, 14]. From the nares, air funnels through two valves, which are the narrowest point of passage. Deformities and the collapse of the alar cartilage can obstruct or stenose the external and internal nasal valves, evaluated by the Cottle test. Between the external and internal nasal valves, septal deviations and enlarged inferior turbinates can further contribute to obstruction of flow. Maxillary constriction and crossbites will further narrow the nasal floor and constrict air flow. The retropalatal area is influenced by the position of the maxilla, soft palate, and adenotonsillar region. A retruded maxilla, decreased space posterior to the hard palate, the thickness and length of the soft palate, lymphoid hyperplasia especially in the adolescent, and certain craniofacial skeletal abnormalities all contribute to airway flow deficiencies. Airway flow can be unintentionally inhibited postsurgically, such as status-post cleft palate repair surgeries or pharyngeal flaps. Chronic OSA has even been shown to cause the palate to thicken, elongate, and descend, further worsening airway flow. The retroglossal region includes the retruded mandible, which pulls the base of the tongue further posterior, obstructing the airway [15]. Lingual tonsillar hypertrophy and a lax epiglottis can also affect the retroglossal or hypopharyngeal airway space. The pharyngeal constrictors mostly function for swallowing; however, some studies show they can minimally contribute to dilation of the upper airway [1], while other studies highly associate the lateral pharyngeal walls with OSA [13, 16]. The relevant musculature associated with OSA is highlighted in Fig. 9.1.

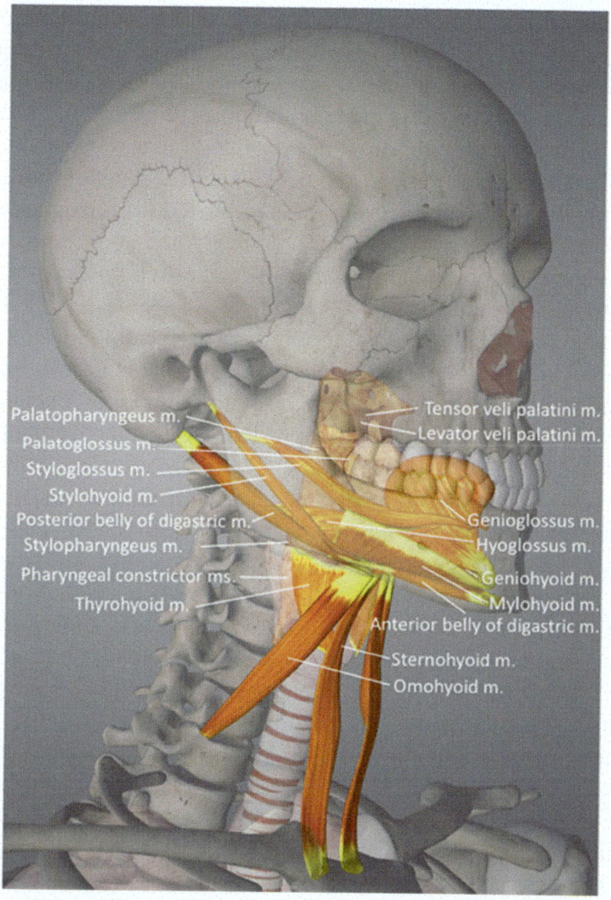

Fig. 9.1 Upper airway muscular anatomy. [Illustration designed by the author using—Essential Anatomy 5, 3D4Medical Limited, Dublin, Ireland]

9.4 Advantages and Indications

Surgical intervention to treat sleep apnea, specifically maxillary and mandibular advancement, can accomplish a myriad of goals, as succinctly delineated in the AAOMS 2017 updated surgical maxillofacial guidelines. Multifactorial indications for surgical intervention seen in the patient's presurgical workup include an elevated Respiratory Disturbance Index (RDI, greater than 20 episodes per hour) or an elevated Apnea-Hypopnea Index (AHI) as measured objectively on polysomnography (PSG), oxygen desaturation <90%, excessive daytime sleepiness (measured subjectively with the Epworth Sleepiness Scale), a positive STOP-BANG questionnaire, failure of medical management, negative esophageal pressures less than 10 cm H_2O, and radiographic evidence of upper airway obstruction and collapse, especially demonstrated with three-dimensional reconstructive airway analyses [2, 15, 17, 18]. Subjectively, a patient could complain of a reduced quality of life, fatigue, snoring, restless nights, and difficulties at work or in relationships, among numerous other chief complaints [2, 15]. On clinical examination, a patient may present with maxillary or mandibular retrognathism, stigmata of craniofacial syndromes, and head and neck anatomical abnormalities or may be obese. Anatomically, surgical intervention is indicated for retrognathia, maxillary hypoplasia, intranasal obstruction, a caudal hyoid bone, macroglossia, an elongated or enlarged soft palate, lymphoid tissue hyperplasia, brachycephaly, and fatty infiltration of the head and neck [13].

A key first step in assessing any intervention is delineating a patient's goals and expectations to evaluate if the goals can realistically be achieved. Reducing AHI, and thus upper airway obstruction and nocturnal hypoxia, is a primary objective goal, but also subjectively reducing daytime sleepiness, improvement in quality of life, and improving cognitive and behavioral function are all chief goals [2, 19]. Surgical intervention can also improve esophageal pressures and pH, as well as improve cardiovascular health and reduce the need for CPAP [2]. The surgical goal is to enlarge the pharyngeal airway via displacement of soft tissues and musculature [15]. Advancement of the mandible anatomically repositions the anterior belly of the digastric, mylohyoid, genioglossus, and geniohyoid muscles, which in turn pulls the tongue superior, anterior, and away from the pharynx to prevent obstruction while also enlarging the retrolingual airway [1, 8]. Advancement of the maxilla enlarges the retropalatal airway by directly pulling the soft tissue of the palate and the palatoglossal muscles anterior and superior, increasing the nasopharyngeal airway, and suspending the tongue forward [1, 8, 20]. Increased activity of the tensor veli palatini, genioglossus, and hyoid musculature appears to increase the airway space and decrease resistance [1]. Maxillary advancement also increases the intranasal airway space by widening the alar base, as well as facilitating the ability to correct any present septal deviation [21]. Limited three-dimensional studies have shown bimaxillary advancement to enlarge the entire velopharynx through elevation of tissues attached to the maxilla, mandible, and hyoid bones [18, 20].

The surgical treatment ladder is controversial. In the literature, some surgeons advocate less invasive surgical interventions with an escalation of treatment in a stepwise fashion from a Phase 1 soft tissue surgical approach to a Phase 2 maxillofacial skeletal surgical procedure, regardless of the anatomical abnormality present. Uvulopalatopharyngoplasty (UPPP) is a viable option in certain cases of mild to moderate OSA to treat retropalatal obstruction but can be more painful and result in unpredictable soft tissue changes and narrowing of the pharyngeal airway [1, 8]. Other surgeons address palatal and base of the tongue anatomical abnormalities first, or in conjunction with MMA, or specifically target a retrolingual obstruction with genioglossus advancement and posterior oropharyngeal obstruction with tonsillectomy and adenoidectomy [1, 22]. In this model, major facial skeletal surgery is only reserved for refractory and/or severe OSA [1]. The controversy lies in the fact that there are minimal surgical parameters that clearly dictate the superior surgical intervention based on each anatomic abnormality with evidence of an improvement in outcome. The anatomical abnormality needs to be treated, as no consistent treatment echelon can be applied to all patients with such a multifactorial disorder [8].

MMA is widely seen to be the most effective surgical approach for multilevel expansion of the upper airway and to significantly reduce AHI [1]. Those that support MMA for moderate to severe OSA, especially OSA refractory to CPAP, as the first intervention, argue that Phase 1 soft tissue surgeries have limited benefit and success and then can actually deter the patient from undergoing further surgery. If MMA is performed first, the patient will experience significant improvement without undergoing multiple procedures [23, 24]. Regardless of the procedure, surgery should target the level of obstruction and the severity of the disorder appropriately [1]. The author recommends strongly considering MMA for the treatment of OSA in patients with moderate to severe OSA and those with craniofacial findings consistent with a propensity for OSA, including mandibular hypoplasia, microgenia, and a narrow maxillary arch.

9.5 Disadvantages, Risks, and Contraindications

The main disadvantages of any surgical intervention stem from improper assessment and planning to treat the anatomic abnormality causing the obstructive sleep apnea. Of course, the same inherent risks of any orthognathic surgery will exist with the MMA procedure, namely, damage to trigeminal nerves, malocclusion, need for prolonged intubation or tracheostomy, immediate failure to improve symptoms, and relapse, among a myriad of other risks [2, 24, 25].

While there are few contraindications to MMA itself, many of the patients with severe OSA often have multiple causally related comorbidities that will put them at increased risk for anesthesia and postoperative complications [2, 26]. A thorough history and physical and detailed discussions with your colleague anesthesiologist can avoid serious perioperative and postoperative sequelae. This topic will be further expounded upon in another chapter.

9.6 Surgical Procedure Overview

The sleep apnea patient necessitating MMA differs from the orthognathic patient due to many factors, including, but not limited to, advanced age and a higher likelihood of multiple comorbidities [15]. While functional improvement with significant advancement is the ultimate goal in MMA, facial aesthetics must still be considered [25, 27]. It has been clearly documented that maxillary and mandibular advancement surgery is very efficacious in resolving OSA by enlarging the pharyngeal airway. This is primarily achieved by pulling the base of the tongue and soft palate anteriorly and tightening the upper airway musculature, namely, the velopharyngeal and suprahyoid muscles, via advancement of their bony origins [3, 9]. MMA can, of course, correct facial and occlusal deformities as well, if planned in conjunction with an orthodontist [3].

Planning an MMA with the goal of function, as well as maintaining or improving aesthetics, can be difficult [8]. Careful discussions with the patient pertaining to ultimate goals are imperative. Radiographic planning with cephalometric films, CBCT, or traditional CT can facilitate either virtual surgical planning (VSP) or traditional model surgery to plan exact movements and to create intraoperative intermediate and final splints (Figs. 9.2 and 9.3) [1, 8, 15, 28, 29]. Radiographically, the airway must be evaluated at multiple levels to deduce the narrowest point of obstruction, to then correlate to the associated anatomical abnormality [1, 15]. Nasopharyngoscopy, either awake or drug-induced sleep endoscopy, should be performed to assist in the evaluation of the anatomical obstruction. However, there is a paucity of data that correlates the method and quality of presurgical evaluations with surgical outcomes [1]. The sequence of surgery should plan for maxillary and then mandibular osteotomies and fixation, with rare exceptions, which should be considered in the fabrication of the intermediate splint [8]. The author prefers the

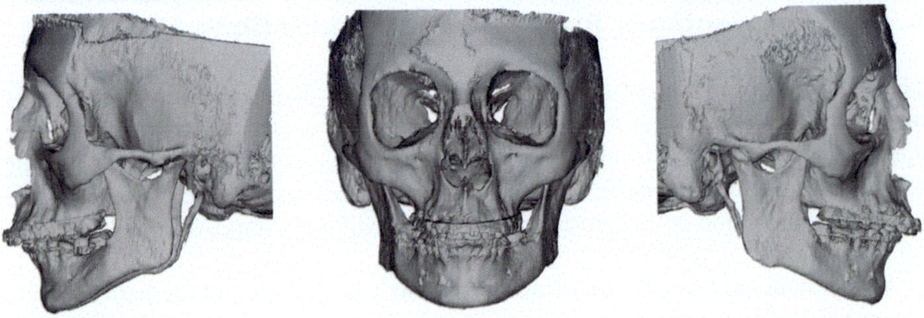

Fig. 9.2 Pre-Operative Virtual Surgical Planning (VSP) Images. VSP allows the surgeon to plan all surgical movements and evaluate and approve the final occlusion, with the ability to present the presurgical outcome to the patient as well

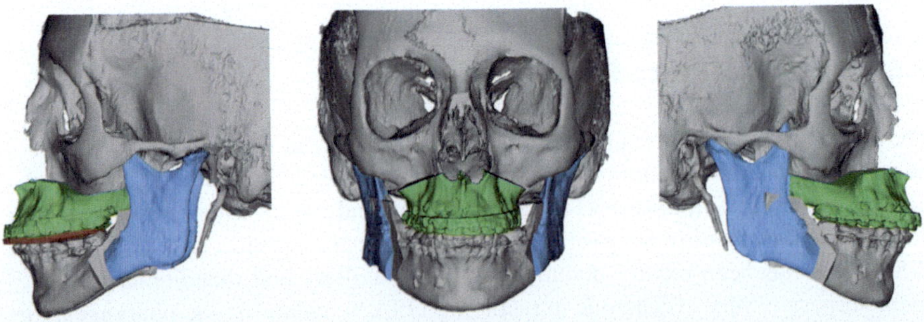

Fig. 9.3 VSP Surgical Plan. This three-dimensional CT rendering illustrates the VSP planned surgical movements, including the final occlusion. The patient can visualize and better understand the surgical procedure, and the surgeon can plan surgical movements to .01 mm, with fabrication of precise occlusal splints

following sequence of progression: (1) genioplasty osteotomies first to free the genioglossus and geniohyoid bearing segment of the anterior mandible; (2) maxillary osteotomies, mobilization, advancement of at least 10 mm, and fixation; (3) bilateral sagittal split mandibular osteotomy (BSSO) and advancement of at least 10 mm with fixation; and (4) finally advancement and fixation of the genioplasty advancement, again of at least 10 mm. The main benefit of completing the genioglossal advancement osteotomy first is that it allows for easier advancement of the mandible without resistance from the genioglossus muscle. Also, the use of a reciprocating saw after fixation of the BSSO advancement may alter or compromise the fixation plates and screws. There is no clear preference in the literature for orthodontic appliances versus intraoperative arch bars for intermaxillary fixation for a functional MMA [1, 22].

Considering that the OSA patient innately has a difficult airway, the patient should not be left wired in MMF postoperatively, further compromising the airway. A nasal RAE endotracheal tube (ETT) is required, as intraoperative MMF is utilized. The endotracheal tube is secured either with a secure headwrap and tape or suturing the ETT to the nasal septum [15]. Based on the difficulty of intubation, postoperative intubation can be considered. This will all be further discussed in the chapter on perioperative airway management. Intraoperatively, close communication with anesthesia is advised. Requesting hypotensive anesthesia (i.e., a mean arterial blood pressure below 60 mmHg) will decrease blood loss during maxillary downfracture while improving visualization. Keeping the patient in a slight reverse Trendelenburg can assist with decreasing blood loss as well [28]. Conservative intravenous fluids will decrease the propensity for postoperative edema and complications [15, 30].

While function is the primary goal of MMA, aesthetic outcome must be considered. MMA is unique from orthognathic surgery in that the typical advancement is 10–12 mm, which runs the risk of excessive over-projection [1, 31]. This should always be discussed with the patient in advance. Unless the patient has a malocclusion that is planned to be corrected, simultaneous mandibular and maxillary advancement should maintain the patient's preoperative occlusion [8, 22].

9.7 Maxillary Surgery

The maxillary advancement in MMA is very similar to the surgical technique utilized in a standard Lefort 1 osteotomy [15, 32]. Pre-incision measurements with a Boley gauge in relation to the maxillary height are important in the MMA patient, as vertical maxillary movements are often not required. Measurements can be made from a K wire placed at nasion or from measurements from the medial canthus bilaterally. Alar base measurements at the beginning of the case and prior to closing help avoid nasal alar base widening.

A horizontal vestibular incision through mucosa from first molar to first molar provides adequate access [15, 22, 32]. The maxilla is then exposed through subperiosteal elevation, extending posteriorly to the pterygoid, anteriorly to the piriform rim, and laterally to the root of the zygoma while preserving the nasal floor mucosa and avoiding excessive retraction of the infraorbital nerve [15, 22, 32]. Hydrodissection with Afrin-soaked pledgets at the nasal floor aids in pushing the mucosal floor superiorly while also providing hemostasis [15]. The horizontal osteotomy is completed with a sagittal or reciprocating saw, at least 5 mm above the apices of the maxillary dentition in a curved pattern, from caudal to cephalad to the piriform aperture. A double guarded nasal osteotome chisels through the ANS and septum, level with the occlusal plane, and aimed caudally. Lateral nasal walls are osteotomized with single-side guarded nasal osteotomes. A curved osteotome fractures the posterior buttress at the pterygomaxillary junction, with a medial and inferior vector. The maxilla is then downfractured and mobilized with Rowe disimpaction forceps, Tessier pterygoid retractors, and/or a bone hook. It is imperative to fully mobilize the maxilla: ensure all bony junctions have been released, and the soft tissue envelope is maximally stretched. The maxillary dentition should fit passively into the intermediate splint with the mandibular condyles seated prior to fixation [15, 22].

Maxillary advancement is routinely 10–12 mm [15, 22]. A rongeur may be required to reduce the ANS with a large advancement in MMA surgery, as this may otherwise cause an obtuse nasolabial angle and over-rotate the nasal tip; again, the goal is often to minimize aesthetic changes while improving function. The nasal apertures can be widened at the base to decrease the degree of alar base widening postoperatively. IMF screws, orthodontic appliances, or arch bars can then be fixated with the intermediate splint, as presurgically planned, to ensure adequate advancement and position of the maxilla [15]. Affirm with a Boley gauge there are no inadvertent vertical changes if none were placed prior to fixation. Fixation should be rigid with large 1.5 mm prebent plates, and fixated with monocortical screws. Zygomaticomaxillary buttresses can be fixated with L- or Z- shaped 1.5 mm plates and monocortical screws. The author also recommends the use and placement of bone grafts (i.e., autograft, allograft, or xenograft), specifically at the anterior maxillary walls bilaterally to help further stabilize the advancement. Figure 9.4 illustrates intraoperative rigid fixation with bone graft placement.

9.8 Mandibular Surgery

Bilateral sagittal split osteotomy (BSSO) is the preferred technique for mandibular advancement. The intraoral incisions bilaterally should be along the external oblique ridge from mid-ramus to lateral of the first molar, subperiosteally elevating the mucosa [15, 22]. While traditionally the medial and lateral border of the mandible were well exposed, the modified sagittal split technique minimizes detachment of the pterygomasseteric sling and periosteum to prevent ischemia and necrosis [15, 22, 33]. While conservatively minimizing medial mandibular detachment, the temporalis muscle should still be stripped from the coronoid process

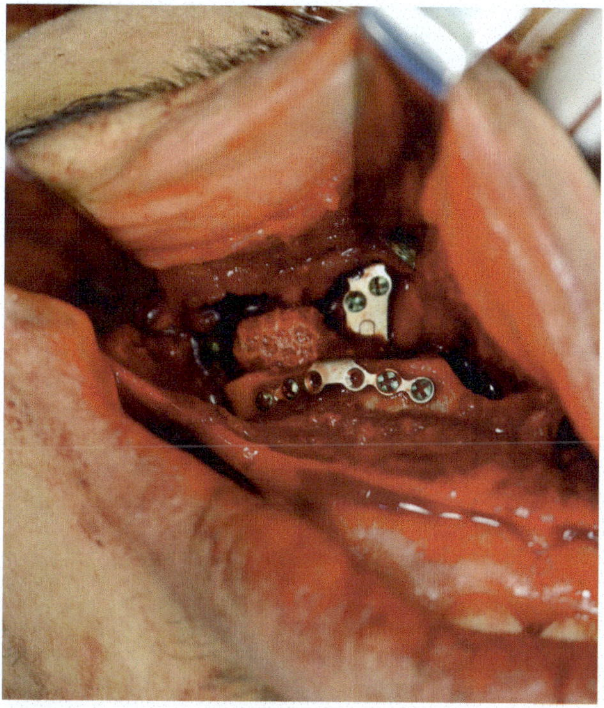

Fig. 9.4 Intraoperative photo depicting maxillary prebent rigid fixation with bone graft placement for increased stability

with a notch retractor to access and identify the lingula [15, 22]. A reciprocating saw is then utilized for the medial monocortical osteotomy, 4–5 mm superior to the foramen while protecting the inferior alveolar nerve, ensuring adequate postero-medial osteotomy to facilitate a favorable split [15, 22]. The monocortical osteotomy with the reciprocating saw can then be continued in a curvilinear fashion along the anterior ramus to the external oblique ridge, 5–6 mm lateral of the molars, to the mesial of the first or second molar to increase the surface area of bony contact. A J stripper and Hargis retractor manipulated in sweeping motions subperiosteally along the mandibular body liberate any muscular attachment, and the lateral osteotomy is then completed with the saw tip from the inferior border of the mandible vertically curving to the osteotomy on the external oblique ridge [15] (Fig. 9.5).

The cortices are split with osteotomes, and carefully used to split the segments with minimal force [22]. The inferior alveolar nerve should be visualized and positioned in the distal (tooth-bearing) segment (Fig. 9.6), and the mandible should be fully mobilized, facilitated by the liberated genioglossus if a genioglossus advancement was completed first [15, 22].

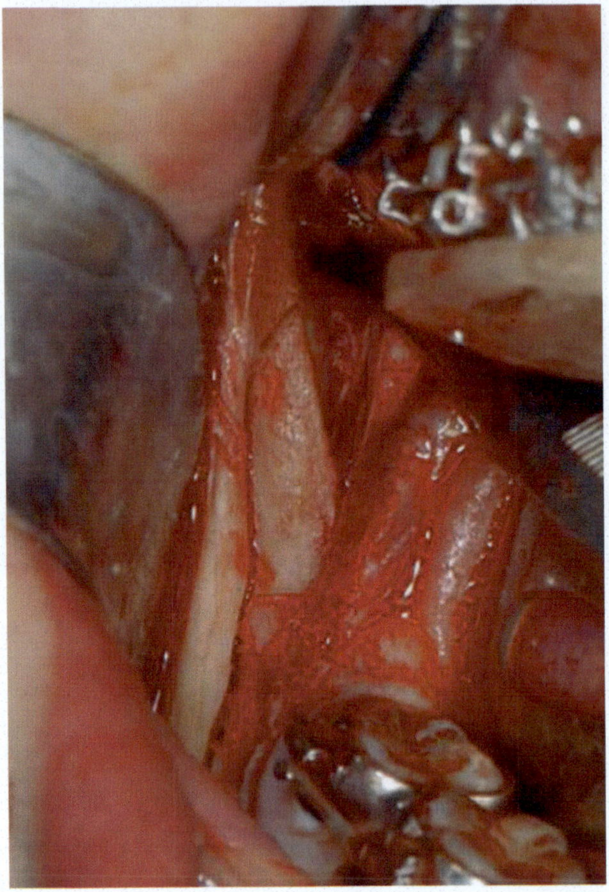

Fig. 9.5 Intraoperative photo depicting the mandibular osteotomies prior to the mandibular split

For final occlusion, a final splint can be used in conjunction with intermaxillary fixation wires [15, 22]. A Jeter-Van Sickels bone clamp holds distal and proximal segments in the desired pre-planned position and compresses the segments while ensuring the inferior borders of the mandibular segments align and the mandibular condyles are well-seated. Rigid fixation via bicortical titanium screws or monocortical plates and screws alone can be sufficient, but as these advancements are often larger than in traditional orthognathic surgery, the combination of both fixation modalities is recommended, especially if the advancement is greater than 7 mm [15, 22, 34]. A slide plate can facilitate a more precise fixation and position of the segments. Transbuccal trocar devices facilitate placement of posterior and positional screw fixation. Advancements can be up to 20 mm, but advancements that large should be considered for distraction osteogenesis secondary to stability [15, 35, 36].

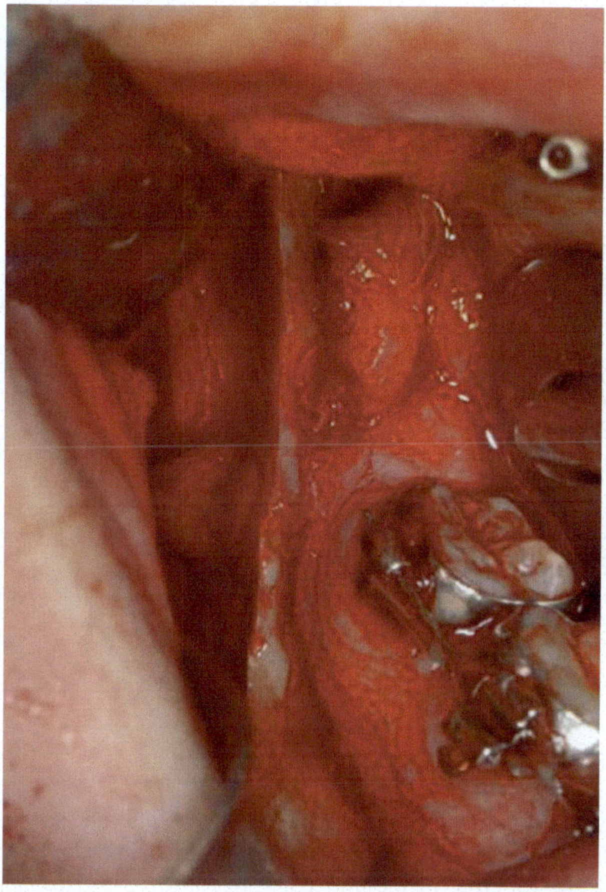

Fig. 9.6 The inferior alveolar nerve remains in the distal (tooth-bearing) segment after the mandibular split (impacted third molar removed simultaneously during osteotomy)

9.9 Genioglossus Advancement

The addition of a genioglossus advancement is often an integral part of MMA surgery, suspending the genioglossus and geniohyoid muscles. This author recommends a true genioglossal advancement rather than a genial tubercle advancement, as this is more stable. While the mobilization of the genioplasty is completed first to facilitate the remainder of the surgery, the fixation with a prebent plate is usually the final step prior to closure. Figure 9.7 illustrates the large genioglossal advancement necessary for optimal postsurgical outcome in the OSA patient. Genial surgery for the treatment of OSA is discussed at length in a dedicated chapter.

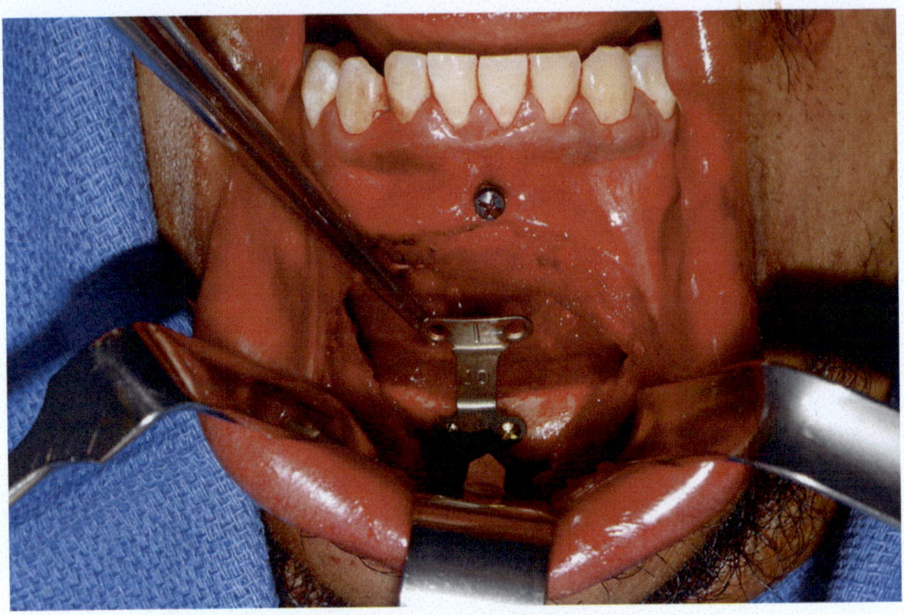

Fig. 9.7 An intraoperative photo depicting a large genioglossal advancement

9.10 Closure

The maxillary vestibular incision closure should include an aesthetic alar cinch suture and single or double V-Y advancement of vestibular tissues to minimize nasal base widening and thinning of the upper lip [1, 15, 33, 37]. The mandibular incisions are closed primarily. The mentalis must be resuspended if a genioglossus advancement was performed. The decision to keep a patient in intermaxillary fixation or in elastics is dependent on the surgeon's experience, but extra precautions must be taken if a patient is kept in maxillomandibular fixation, due to the postoperative airway risks, and thus elastics are preferred [15, 22].

9.11 Post-operative Care

In contrast to the usual young and healthy orthognathic patient, the severe OSA patient necessitating MMA surgery complicates postoperative medical management. Airway is the chief concern in this population, and sedating analgesics further decreases pharyngeal tone and arousal response to hypoxia, resulting in obstruction and hypercarbia. Patient-controlled analgesia (PCA) should be avoided, and pain should instead be managed with small IV doses and longer-acting oral medications, with continuous monitoring of respiratory rates and oxygenation [13, 15]. IV dexamethasone intraoperatively and postoperatively reduces edema [22]. PAP should not be used postoperatively, as this can lead to significant subcutaneous emphysema. Bleeding complications can be reduced with strict blood pressure control, maintaining the MAP approximately 90–100 with aggressive antihypertensives. Diet should be conservative with large advancements concerning for stability, progressing from liquids to a soft diet for 6 weeks [15, 22].

Follow-up is dependent on the patient's postoperative course and surgeon preference. The patient should be counseled on beginning CPAP therapy at 6 weeks postoperatively, with continued use for 4–6 months, until a postoperative polysomnogram is performed [15, 22, 38].

9.12 Surgical Complications

Hypoesthesia, dysesthesia, and paresthesia rates vary in the literature. The prevalence of immediate postoperative facial hypoesthesia is nearly guaranteed, but a study of 40 patients showed 12.5% persistent long-term anesthesia of the inferior alveolar nerve, while another meta-analysis found paresthesia to persist in 14.2% [39, 40]. More rare complications include severe bleeding, hematoma, malocclusion, TMJ derangement, infection necessitating hardware removal, instability of the maxilla, and relapse [1, 8, 26]. If the OSA patient is inappropriately medically managed, the sequelae can be very serious: reintubation, prolonged hospitalization, cardiovascular events, and even death. Proper preoperative assessment and patient selection, as well as perioperative and postoperative management as discussed above, may lessen the risk. Airway complications perioperatively and postoperatively in the first 72 hours can be grave and will be further discussed in another chapter [1, 4, 13, 26].

9.13 Alternative Surgical Approaches

Similar to distraction osteogenesis (DO) in the pediatric patient with craniofacial abnormalities, this procedure should be considered when advancements necessitated are over 1 cm and reaching 2 cm [15]. Outcomes appear to be comparable for smaller advancements compared to BSSO, but DO may be advantageous for advancements over 7 mm, although there is a paucity of clinical trials [41]. Distraction in this population can achieve 1 mm per day without a latency period, with possible need for bone grafting [15].

Other alternatives to BSSO and DO exist, such as inverted L- or C- osteotomies of the mandibular rami. These osteotomies can be performed through both transoral or transcervical approaches and generally require bone grafting and fixation with locking reconstruction plates with large advancements. These osteotomies are generally reserved for reoperation cases and/or patient's with abnormal mandibular anatomy.

9.14 Outcomes

A key first step in deciding any intervention is delineating patient goals and expectations. The challenge of any facial surgery is that both function and aesthetics must always be considered and compromised.

Surgical outcome is both subjective and objective. Subjective surveys such as the Epworth sleepiness scale preoperatively and surveys of aesthetics and quality of life changes postoperatively can define patient satisfaction [27, 31, 42–44]. The surgeon and sleep medicine physician will often focus on more objective parameter outcomes to define surgical success. The American Academy of Sleep Medicine standardizes Apnea-Hypopnea Index (AHI, as detailed in previous chapters) with polysomnography repeat studies as an objective classifier, and thus AHI can be a primary endpoint in evaluating the different surgical approaches [1].

CPAP is the gold standard of care in OSA, but the elimination of the need for CPAP is a common goal of surgery and a clear objective success. Most patients postoperatively no longer require CPAP, with one study demonstrating that 93% of patients discontinue use [1, 8]. Other studies revealed success through polysomnographic studies with decreased respiratory disturbance index (RDI) outcomes, decreased oxygen desaturation while sleeping, and an increase in stage 3, 4, and REM sleep cycles [22, 45]. The American Academy of Sleep Medicine meta-analysis of nine studies of patients with severe OSA undergoing MMA consistently and significantly reduced AHI, achieving an average AHI decrease from 54.5 to 7.7, which is an 87% decrease compared with UPPP, which reduced AHI by only 33% [46]. Another meta-analysis of 22 studies and 627 patients undergoing MMA found the mean AHI to decrease from 63.9 to 9.5 at an average 5-month follow-up [40]. A long-term follow-up study over an average 4.2 years of 40 patients revealed a significant continued reduction in RDI, averaging 71.2 preoperatively to an average of 7.6 in long-term follow-up [39]. Interestingly, when developing an early surgical protocol, Riley et al. staged 239 patients for UPPP and found 24 patients progressed to MMA surgery after failed UPPP for severe OSA and then achieved a 100% surgical success rate with MMA [9].

With the improvement in imaging, three-dimensional volumetric analyses comparing presurgical and postsurgical upper airway changes may become the gold standard objective outcome assessment (Figs. 9.8 and 9.9). MMA increases the total airway volume, specifically the retropalatal and retrolingual airway volumes [18, 47].

Although subjective outcomes are more difficult to quantify, they can often be more significant to the patient than objective successes. In multiple studies, MMA compared to UPPP achieved a decrease in Epworth sleepiness scores, depressive symptoms, and pain while reporting a high level of satisfaction and improved cosmesis [8, 22]. Multiple smaller case studies aggregately supported improved sleep quality, quality of life,

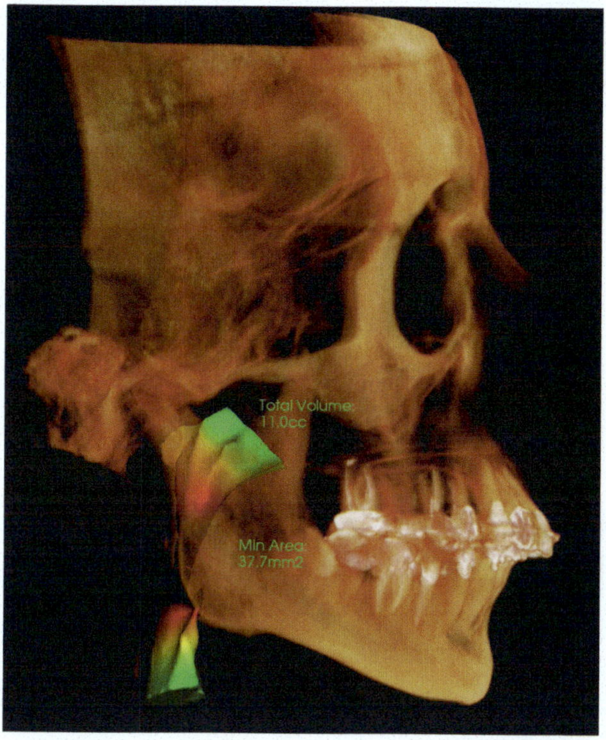

Fig. 9.8 Pre-operative three-dimensional airway volume analysis. [Software—Invivo6, Anatomage, San Jose, CA]

headaches, snoring, memory loss, difficulty concentrating, and mood [23, 48]. Aesthetically, patients appear to be largely pleased with the outcome. In multiple studies, the majority of patients saw favorable aesthetic changes, and a large portion of the remainder felt neutral, while under 10% were dissatisfied with the aesthetic changes [39, 43, 48].

9.15 Summary

Maxillary and mandibular advancement surgery is a reliable and successful treatment for moderate to severe obstructive sleep apnea. The surgeon should openly discuss surgical goals and outcomes with the patient prior to proceeding with surgery, as this surgery is not without risks and possible changes in facial aesthetic appearance. Nonetheless, this procedure can lead to immediate and life-changing improvements to a chronic disease.

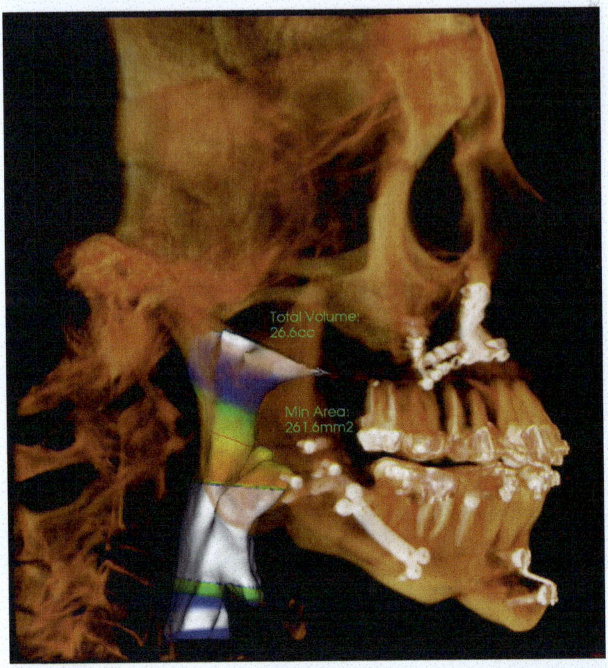

Fig. 9.9 Six-month postoperative three-dimensional airway volume analysis, showing significant objective improvement in airway volume. [Software—Invivo6, Anatomage, San Jose, CA]

References

1. Garg RK, Afifi AM, Sanchez R, King TW. Obstructive sleep apnea in adults: the role of upper airway and facial skeletal surgery. Plast Reconstr Surg. 2016;138:889.
2. Cottrell DA, Farrell B, Ferrer-Nuin L, Ratner S. Surgical correction of maxillofacial skeletal deformities. J Oral Maxillofac Surg. 2017;75:e94.
3. Mehra P, Wolford LM. Surgical management of obstructive sleep apnea. Proc (Bayl Univ Med Cent). 2000;13:338.
4. Esclamado RM, Glenn MG, McCulloch TM, Cummings CW. Perioperative complications and risk factors in the surgical treatment of obstructive sleep apnea syndrome. Laryngoscope. 1989;99:1125.
5. Epstein LJ, Kristo D, Strollo PJ, Friedman N, Malhotra A, Patil SP, Ramar K, Rogers R, Schwab RJ, Weaver EM, Weinstein MD. Adult obstructive sleep apnea task force of the American Academy of Sleep Medicine: clinical guideline for the evaluation, management and long-term care of obstructive sleep apnea in adults. J Clin Sleep Med. 2009;5:263.
6. Aurora RN, Casey KR, Kristo D, Auerbach S, Bista SR, Chowdhuri S, Karippot A, Lamm C, Ramar K, Zak R, Morgenthaler TI, American Academy of Sleep Medicine. Practice parameters for the surgical modifications of the upper airway for obstructive sleep apnea in adults. Sleep. 2010;33:1408.
7. Kapur VK, Auckley DH, Chowdhuri S, Kuhlmann DC, Mehra R, Ramar K, Harrod CG. Clinical practice guideline for diagnostic testing for adult obstructive sleep apnea: an American Academy of Sleep Medicine clinical practice guideline. J Clin Sleep Med. 2017;13(3):479–504.

8. Goodday R. Diagnosis, treatment planning, and surgical correction of obstructive sleep apnea. J Oral Maxillofac Surg. 2009;67:2183.
9. Riley RW, Powell NB, Guilleminault C. Obstructive sleep apnea syndrome: a surgical protocol for dynamic upper airway reconstruction. J Oral Maxillofac Surg. 1993;51:742.
10. Fujita S, Conway W, Zorick F, Roth T. Surgical correction of anatomic abnormalities in obstructive sleep apnea syndrome: uvulopalatopharyngoplasty. Otolaryngol Head Neck Surg. 1981;89:923.
11. Simmons FB, Guilleminault C, Miles LE. The palatopharyngoplasty operation for snoring and sleep apnea: an interim report. Otolaryngol Head Neck Surg. 1984;92:375.
12. Conway W, Fujita S, Zorick F, Sicklesteel J, Roehrs T, Wittig R, Roth T. Uvulopalatopharyngoplasty. One-year follow-up. Chest. 1985;88:385.
13. Porhomayon J, El-Solh A, Chhangani S, Nader ND. The management of surgical patients with obstructive sleep apnea. Lung. 2011;189:359.
14. Schendel S. The airway assessment of the patient with obstructive sleep apnea. In: McNamara J, editor. Surgical enhancement of orthodontic treatment, vol. 47. Ann Arbor: University of Michigan; 2009. p. 203–30.
15. Schendel S, Powell N, Jacobson R. Maxillary, mandibular, and chin advancement: treatment planning based on airway anatomy in obstructive sleep apnea. J Oral Maxillofac Surg. 2011;69:663.
16. Schellenberg JB, Maislin G, Schwab RJ. Physical findings and the risk for obstructive sleep apnea. Am J Respir Crit Care Med. 2000;162:740.
17. Zinser MJ, Zachow S, Sailer HF. Bimaxillary "rotation advancement" procedures in patients with obstructive sleep apnea: a 3-dimensional airway analysis of morphological changes. Int J Oral Maxillofac Surg. 2013;42:569.
18. Louro RS, Calasans-Maia JA, Mattos CT, Masterson D, Calasans-Maia MD, Maia LC. Three-dimensional changes to the upper airway after maxillomandibular advancement with counterclockwise rotation: a systematic review and meta-analysis. Int J Oral Maxillofac Surg. 2018;47:622.
19. Butterfield KJ, Marks PL, McLean L, Newton J. Quality of life assessment after maxillomandibular advancement surgery for obstructive sleep apnea. J Oral Maxillofac Surg. 2016;74:1228.
20. Fairburn SC, Waite PD, Vilos G, Harding SM, Bernreuter W, Cure J, Cherala S. Three-dimensional changes in upper airways of patients with obstructive sleep apnea following maxillomandibular advancement. J Oral Maxillofac Surg. 2007;65:6.
21. Posnick JC, Choi E, Adachie A, Troost T. Correction of symptomatic chronic nasal airway obstruction in conjunction with bimaxillary orthognathic surgery: does it complicate recovery and is it effective? J Oral Maxillofac Surg. 2016;74:620.e1.
22. Hester JE, Powell NB, Riley RW, Li KK. Maxillary-mandibular advancement for obstructive sleep apnea. Oper Tech Otolaryngol Head Neck Surg. 2002;13:135.
23. Hochban W, Conradt R, Brandenburg U, Heitmann J, Peter JH. Surgical maxillofacial treatment of obstructive sleep apnea. Plast Reconstr Surg. 1997;99:618.
24. Zaghi S, Holty JE, Certal V, Abdullatif J, Guilleminault C, Powell NB, Riley RW, Camacho M. Maxillomandibular advancement for treatment of obstructive sleep apnea: a meta-analysis. JAMA Otolaryngol Head Neck Surg. 2016;142:58.
25. Tiner BD, Waite PD. Surgical and nonsurgical management of obstructive sleep apnea. In: Miloro M, Ghali G, Larsen P, Waite P, editors. Principles of oral and maxillofacial surgery. 2nd ed. Hamilton: BC Decker Inc; 2004. p. 1297–313.
26. Posnick JC, Choi E, Chavda A. Operative time, airway management, need for blood transfusions, and in-hospital stay for bimaxillary, intranasal, and osseous genioplasty surgery: current clinical practices. J Oral Maxillofac Surg. 2016;74:590.
27. Islam S, Aleem F, Ormiston IW. Subjective assessment of facial aesthetics after maxillofacial orthognathic surgery for obstructive sleep apnoea. Br J Oral Maxillofac Surg. 2015;53:235.
28. Perciaccante V, Bays R. Bimaxillary orthognathic surgery. In: Kademani D, Tiwana P, editors. Atlas of oral and maxillofacial surgery. 1st ed. St. Louis: Elsevier Inc; 2016. p. 426–34.

29. Teitelbaum J, Diminutto M, Comiti S, Pepin JL, Deschaux C, Raphael B, Bettega G. Lateral cephalometric radiography of the upper airways for evaluation of surgical treatment of obstructive sleep apnea syndrome. Rev Stomatol Chir Maxillofac. 2007;108:13.
30. Ettinger KS, Wyles CC, Bezak BJ, Yildirim Y, Arce K, Viozzi CF. Impact of perioperative fluid administration on postoperative morbidity and length of hospital stay following maxillomandibular advancement for obstructive sleep apnea. J Oral Maxillofac Surg. 2015;73:1372.
31. Ahn HW, Cho IS, Cho KC, Choi JY, Chung JW, Baek SH. Surgical treatment modality for facial esthetics in an obstructive sleep apnea patient with protrusive upper lip and acute nasolabial angle. Angle Orthod. 2013;83:355.
32. Schendel SA, Powell NB. Surgical orthognathic management of sleep apnea. J Craniofac Surg. 2007;18:902.
33. Bell WH, Schendel SA. Biologic basis for modification of the sagittal ramus split operation. J Oral Surg. 1977;35(5):362–9.
34. Ronchi P, Cinquini V, Ambrosoli A, Caprioglio A. Maxillomandibular advancement in obstructive sleep apnea syndrome patients: a retrospective study on the sagittal cephalometric variables. J Oral Maxillofac Res. 2013;4:e5.
35. Bouchard C, Troulis MJ, Kaban LB. Management of obstructive sleep apnea: role of distraction osteogenesis. Oral Maxillofac Surg Clin North Am. 2009;21:459.
36. Lee SH, Kaban LB, Lahey ET. Skeletal stability of patients undergoing maxillomandibular advancement for treatment of obstructive sleep apnea. J Oral Maxillofac Surg. 2015;73:694.
37. Schendel SA, Carlotti AE. Nasal considerations in orthognathic surgery. Am J Orthod Dentofac Orthop. 1991.
38. Riley R, Powell NB, Guilleminault C. Obstructive sleep apnea surgery: risk management and complications. Otolaryngol Head Neck Surg. 1997;117:648.
39. Riley RW, Powell NB, Li KK, Troell RJ, Guilleminault C. Surgery and obstructive sleep apnea: long-term clinical outcomes. Otolaryngol Head Neck Surg. 2000;122:415.
40. Holty JE, Guilleminault C. Maxillomandibular advancement for the treatment of obstructive sleep apnea: a systematic review and meta-analysis. Sleep Med Rev. 2010;14:287.
41. Schreuder WHH, Jansma J, Bierman MW, Vissink A. Distraction osteogenesis versus bilateral sagittal split osteotomy for advancement of the retrognathic mandible: a review of the literature. Int J Oral Maxillofac Surg. 2007.
42. Goodday R, Gregoire C. Facial appearance following surgical treatment for obstructive sleep apnea syndrome. Gen Dent. 2008;56:251.
43. Li KK, Riley RW, Powell NB, Guilleminault C. Patient's perception of the facial appearance after maxillomandibular advancement for obstructive sleep apnea syndrome. J Oral Maxillofac Surg. 2001;59:371.
44. Cohen-Levy J, Petelle B, Vieille E, Dumitrache M, Fleury B. Changes in facial profile after maxillomandibular advancement surgery for obstructive sleep apnea syndrome. Int Orthod. 2013;11:71.
45. Liu SYC, Huon LK, Ruoff C, Riley RW, Strohl KP, Peng Z. Restoration of sleep architecture after maxillomandibular advancement: success beyond the apnea–hypopnea index. Int J Oral Maxillofac Surg. 2017;46:1533.
46. Caples SM, Rowley JA, Prinsell JR, Pallanch JF, Elamin MB, Katz SG, Harwick JD. Surgical modifications of the upper airway for obstructive sleep apnea in adults: a systematic review and meta-analysis. Sleep. 2010;33:1396.
47. Christovam IO, Lisboa CO, Ferreira DMTP, Cury-Saramago AA, Mattos CT. Upper airway dimensions in patients undergoing orthognathic surgery: a systematic review and meta-analysis. Int J Oral Maxillofac Surg. 2016;45(4):460–71.
48. Prinsell JR. Maxillomandibular advancement surgery in a site-specific treatment approach for obstructive sleep apnea in 50 consecutive patients. Chest. 1999;116:1519.

Operative Airway Management and Tracheostomy

10

Anthony M. Bunnell and Rui P. Fernandes

10.1 Introduction

Tracheostomy is a commonly performed procedure for many indications including complex maxillofacial trauma, head and neck oncologic resections, airway obstruction, need for prolonged ventilator support, and obstructive sleep apnea. Tracheostomy used for treatment of obstructive sleep apnea was first described by Kuhlo et al. in 1969 [1]. Tracheostomies were performed as the main surgical therapy for obstructive sleep apnea in patients failing medical therapy well into the early 1980s until the advent of CPAP [2]. This was followed by the introduction of other surgical interventions including uvulopalatopharyngoplasty, hypopharyngeal surgery, and maxillomandibular advancement, which led to a significant change in management strategies for these patients.

While tracheostomy is often considered the last resort in the treatment of OSA, it remains a viable option in those who have failed medical management, are not surgical candidates, or refuse other surgical modalities [3]. Tracheostomy achieves successful resolution of OSA because it completely bypasses any source of upper airway obstruction. A meta-analysis by Camacho et al. [2] has shown that tracheostomy significantly decreases apnea index, oxygen desaturation index, sleepiness, and mortality in patients with OSA. It has been shown to improve and may extend the life of patients with severe OSA [4]. It can quickly reverse associated cardiovascular comorbid conditions including arrhythmias, pulmonary hypertension, and hypoxia [5, 6]. Multiple studies have suggested that aggressive treatment of OSA improves overall survival [4, 7, 8].

Patients with OSA raise concerns regarding the technical difficulty in performing tracheostomy due to differences in anatomy. These variations include difficulty

A. M. Bunnell (✉) · R. P. Fernandes
Division of Head and Neck Surgery, Department of Oral and Maxillofacial Surgery, College of Medicine, University of Florida—Jacksonville, Jacksonville, FL, USA
e-mail: anthony.bunnell@jax.ufl.edu; rui.fernandes@jax.ufl.edu

S. O. Salman (ed.), *Modern Management of Obstructive Sleep Apnea*,
https://doi.org/10.1007/978-3-030-11443-5_10

palpating anterior neck landmarks, shortened neck, excessive submental and upper thoracic tissue obstructing the surgical field, and thickness of structures overlying the trachea. The standard tracheostomy tube curvature may not conform to these anatomical differences [9]. They are often too short and too curved making them more difficult to place and more likely to become dislodged. Dislodgement of these poorly fitting tracheostomy tubes has been associated with increased morbidity and mortality [10].

These patients are often obese, as obesity is considered a major risk factor for development and progression of OSA [11]. In the adult population, the prevalence of OSA is estimated to range from 25 to 45% of obese patients [11–17]. This prevalence of OSA in obese or morbidly obese patients is nearly twice that of normal weight adults [18]. Soft tissue and skeletal surgeries for OSA are less successful in patients who are morbidly obese, and tracheostomy has demonstrated effectiveness in morbidly obese patients [19].

While the perioperative complication rate of tracheostomy among adults ranges in the literature from 4 to 40% [18], open tracheostomy in the OSA patient (obese or nonobese) presents specific challenges that can increase the overall morbidity and mortality of this operation. These challenges can be managed with modifications of the surgical technique and proper tracheostomy tube selection. The goal of the procedure is to provide a safe and effective airway that will require minimal postoperative care.

10.2 Perioperative Management

Regardless of planned surgical intervention, proper preoperative medical optimization is crucial when treating patients with OSA. The comorbidities associated with OSA are well documented and should be managed preoperatively to minimize complications. CPAP should be used in the preoperative period and, depending on surgical intervention, postoperatively as well. For some procedures, such as maxillomandibular advancement, CPAP should be avoided postoperatively due to risk of head and neck subcutaneous emphysema. In terms of medical optimization, hypertension, cardiovascular disease, and diabetes should all be optimized and well controlled prior to surgery.

Airway management and plan should be discussed with the anesthesia team in detail prior to surgery. Patients with OSA innately have difficult airways and may be challenging intubations. Adjuncts such as fiber-optic scopes and video intubation scopes should be available and utilized if needed. The surgical team should also be prepared for possible awake tracheostomy.

Regarding anesthetic care, long-acting sedative and opioid agents should be limited. Anesthetic agents promote pharyngeal collapse, reduce ventilation, blunt respiratory response to carbon dioxide, and blunt arousal from sleep. Patients with OSA have a higher sensitivity to opioids, benzodiazepines, and other sedative agents. Central opioid receptors are upregulated in patients with OSA due to recurrent hypoxia [20]; therefore, smaller doses should be used. Prior to extubation, full reversal from muscle relaxation should be confirmed.

Postoperatively, opioids and other sedative agents should be minimized, as they are the leading causes of adverse outcomes postoperatively [21, 22]. Other adjuncts, such as acetaminophen, corticosteroids, tramadol, topical agents, gabapentin/pregabalin, etc., should be used instead. Blood pressure control is essential as well, especially with base of tongue, tracheal, tonsillar, and maxillary advancement surgery to prevent postoperative bleeding. Postsurgical OSA patients should be monitored in either an intensive care or progressive (step-down) unit setting for closer observation.

10.3 Surgical Technique

Open tracheostomy is performed under general anesthesia in the operating room for the OSA patient regardless of body habitus. For the obese patient, considerable time and effort are often required to transfer and position the patient in a safe and appropriate manner [23]. To assist operating room personnel with transfer of the patient to the operating room table, a HoverMatt Air Transfer System (HoverTech International, Bethlehem, PA) is used (Fig. 10.1). Often the patient's excess submental adipose and chest tissues are retracted from the neck surgical site using foam pads and silk tape. Excess adipose tissue between the sternum and trachea will cause a posterior inferior slant of the trachea. These patients may also have a short neck displacing the airway further inferiorly into the chest. Placement of a shoulder roll and neck extension will allow for maximum exposure to the anterior neck and surgical field (Fig. 10.2).

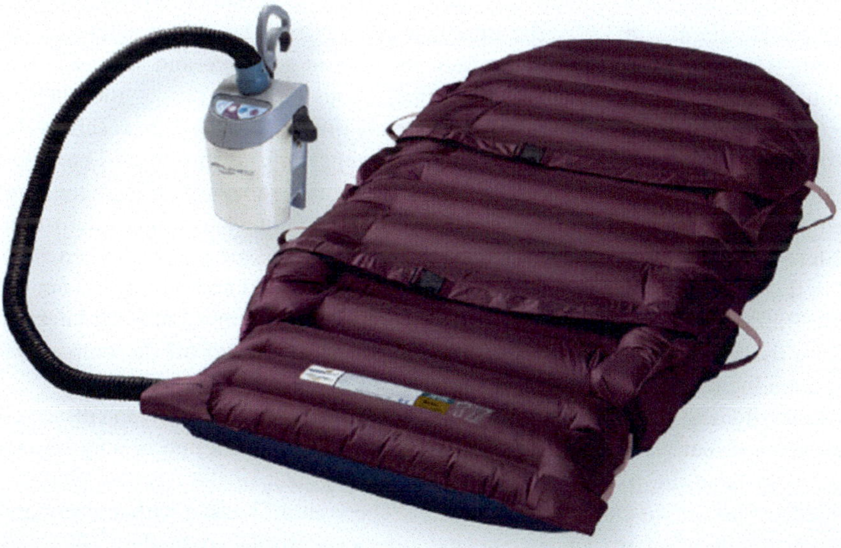

Fig. 10.1 HoverMatt® Air Transfer System (HoverTech International, Bethlehem, PA)

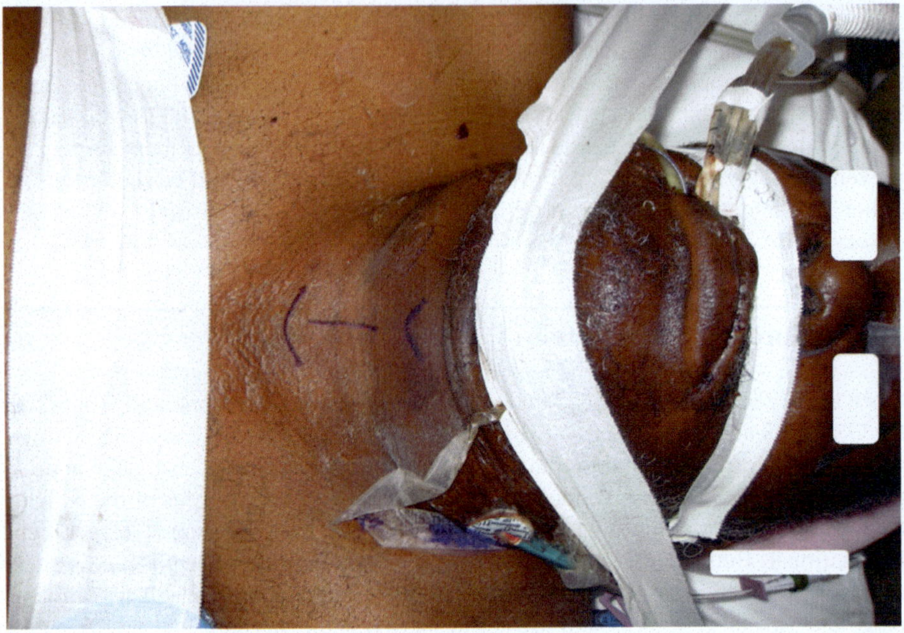

Fig. 10.2 Taping and positioning of the obese patient to provide maximum exposure of the anterior neck and surgical field

As in a standard open tracheostomy, all surgical landmarks are identified prior to incision. These landmarks include the sternal notch, cricoid, and thyroid cartilages. For the obese patient with OSA, the authors prefer a horizontal skin incision 3–4 cm in length. This is placed midway between the cricoid cartilage and sternal notch. Incision is made through the skin and subcutaneous tissue exposing the anterior cervical adipose tissue. A lipectomy in this area is often needed before reaching the platysma. Subplatysmal flaps are then elevated superiorly to the thyroid cartilage and inferiorly to the sternal notch. The anterior jugular veins are encountered and ligated and divided bilaterally. This helps minimize untimely bleeding later in the procedure or postoperatively. Additional excess adipose tissue that is now encountered in the central compartment of the neck is then elevated and removed from the deeper strap muscles. The strap muscles are then separated and retracted laterally exposing the thyroid isthmus. The thyroid isthmus is dissected off the pretracheal fascia, then ligated, divided, and tied with 2-0 silk sutures.

With the thyroid gland now retracted laterally, the pretracheal fascia is dissected off, allowing direct visualization of the upper trachea. Two traction or stay sutures using 2-0 Prolene are placed through the anterior aspect of the tracheal rings on either side of the site of entry into the trachea. These sutures assist with anterior and cephalad mobilization of a posterior and inferiorly displaced trachea. The stay sutures are left in place postoperatively for 1–2 weeks to assist in replacement of the tracheostomy tube in case of inadvertent dislodgement or decannulation. If needed, a tracheal hook can also be used to mobilize the trachea in a cephalad direction, bringing the trachea closer to the skin surface. A vertical or horizontal incision is made within the trachea in between the second and third tracheal ring. The opening is dilated and the endotracheal tube is withdrawn. For planned lifelong tracheostomy use, an alternative option is removal or excision of the anterior aspect of 1–2 tracheal rings, providing a much larger opening. A cuffed tracheostomy tube (tube selection discussed later in this chapter) is then inserted into the airway trachea and connected to the anesthesia circuit. Assessment for end-tidal carbon dioxide and appropriate tidal volumes is completed, and the endotracheal tube is then completely removed. It is our practice to secure the tracheostomy tube to the skin with silk sutures for the initial postoperative period until the tube is changed.

10.4 Tracheostomy Tube Selection

There are a number of clinical and technical considerations associated with tracheostomy tube selection. The anatomical differences listed previously, including a posterior and inferiorly displaced airway, may not allow for use of a standard tracheostomy tube. This may necessitate the use of a Shiley™ extended-length tracheostomy tube (Medtronic, Minneapolis, MN). These are available in either proximal (Fig. 10.3) or distal extensions (Fig. 10.4). The proximal extension refers to the distance between the flange and bend of the tube accounting for the increased thickness of the anterior neck. The distal extension refers to the distance after the bend to the tip of the tube, which may assist with an inferiorly displaced trachea. Other

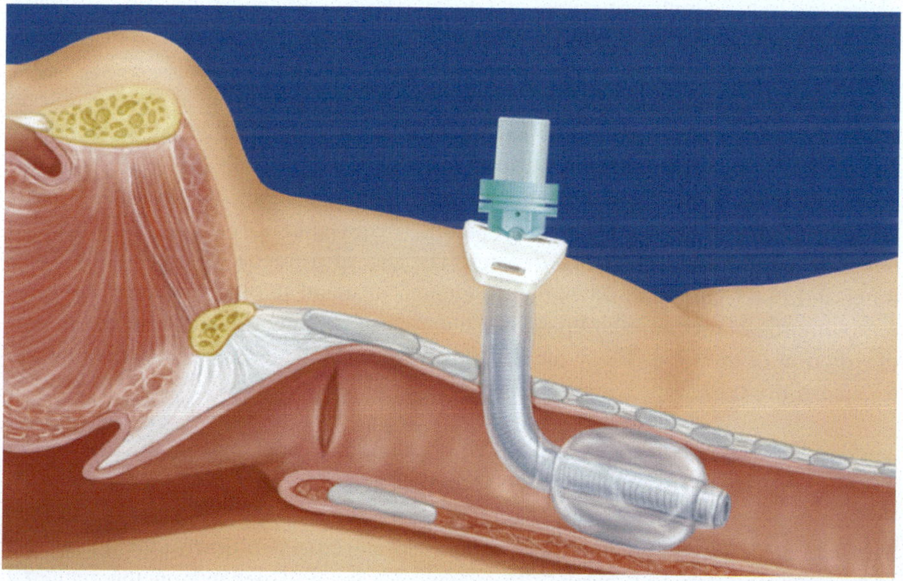

Fig. 10.3 Shiley™ tracheostomy tube with proximal extension (Medtronic, Minneapolis, MN)

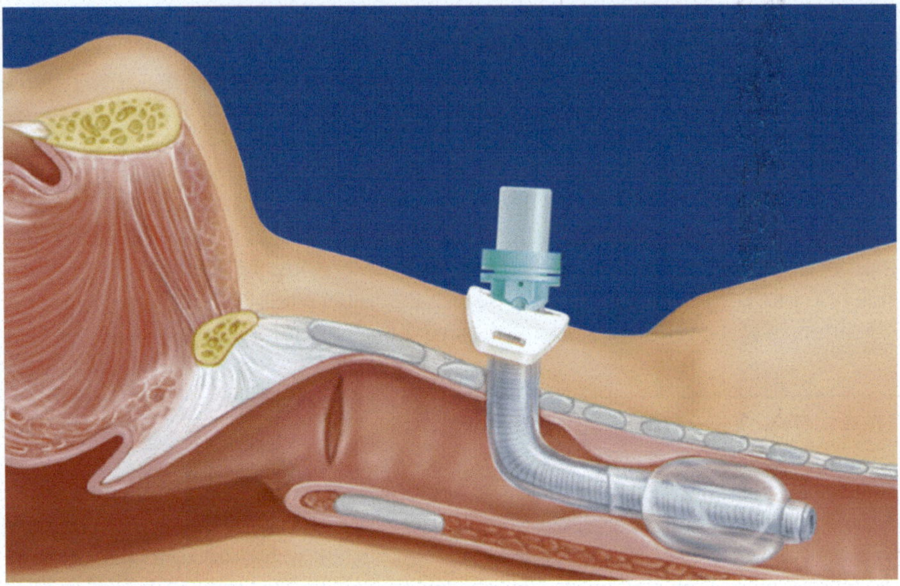

Fig. 10.4 Shiley™ tracheostomy tube with distal extension (Medtronic, Minneapolis, MN)

anatomical differences may include unanticipated significant tracheal deviation or stenosis that may be encountered during dissection or upon entering the airway. Tracheal deviation or stenosis may complicate placement, but this can be circumvented with placement of a distally extended tracheostomy tube. It is the authors' preference to have both a proximal and distal extension tracheostomy tube available until the airway is encountered surgically to determine which tube is most appropriate.

In addition to anatomical differences of the airway, other clinical considerations when selecting the correct tracheostomy tube include ventilation needs, need for supplemental oxygen, ambulation and activity needs, speech, and feeding concerns. Technical considerations include tube brand availability, need for a cuff, need for fenestration, need for inner cannula (disposable or reusable), and need to integrate with other respiratory devices. The use of a tracheostomy tube with an inner and outer cannula allows one to change or clean the inner cannula without removing the outer cannula. Frequent changing of the inner cannula helps prevent obstruction of the tube. These factors must also be considered prior to placing the tracheostomy tube.

10.5 Postoperative Tracheostomy Care

The patient is monitored in either an intensive care or step-down unit during the immediate postoperative period. The level of care will depend on the patient's comorbidities, experience of nursing staff, and bed or unit availability. Regardless of the level of care, the nursing staff should be familiar with all aspects of tracheostomy care. This allows for nursing staff to also help educate the patient and family members with tracheostomy care. Routine care includes the need for humidification and frequent suctioning to prevent mucous plugging and airway obstruction. It is encouraged to begin educating the patient and family on the first day so they feel comfortable with routine care at the time of discharge.

There is no accepted standard for adult tracheostomy tube changes, and most tracheostomy tube exchange protocols are a result of institutional practices. If the patient does not require positive-pressure ventilation, the tube can be typically changed to a fenestrated uncuffed tube on the third postoperative day after the track is well defined. The patient is discharged with the necessary equipment to replace the inner cannula, clean the stoma, and manage the wound. They should be proficient in tube removal and insertion so they can manage a mucous plug if necessary. Common home care tracheostomy and stoma cleaning agents include hydrogen peroxide, commercial medical disinfectants, and simple soap and water. When the patient is discharged home, often one tracheostomy care cleaning kit is utilized once daily for stoma site cleaning and care. Patients are sent home once the nursing staff are confident with the patient and/or family's ability to manage the tracheostomy tube.

Regular office visits are necessary in the first 6 months in order to remove or cauterize any stomal granulation tissue. This can occur anywhere in the stoma but is most common at the superior edge of the stoma. Despite removing anterior cervical adipose tissue during tracheostomy, the distance from the trachea to the skin remains long. The tracheostomy ties pull superiorly because of the short neck and tend to worsen granulation tissue at the superior aspect of the stoma. Silver nitrate is quick and effective in removing or shrinking granulation tissue. Electrocautery is more effective for larger lesions but will require a return to the operating room.

There is, however, a subset of morbidly obese patients who may have additional requirements for ventilator support in order to improve daytime symptoms and nocturnal ventilation. Reasons for lack of improvement in obese patients include obstruction of the tracheostomy tube by redundant soft tissue, kinking of the tracheostomy tube, displacement of the tracheostomy tube, or the patients may have comorbid obesity hypoventilation syndrome [19].

Polysomnography (with CO_2 monitoring as appropriate) to assess surgical effectiveness of tracheostomy for OSA can be performed to rule out postoperative central apneas, hypopneas, and/or obesity hypoventilation syndrome that could warrant positive airway pressure therapy through the tracheostomy [18, 19].

The time frame to decannulation varies widely among patients. Decannulation process typically involves a sequential downsizing of the tube followed by capping trials if the patient can tolerate it. Reasons for decannulation include intolerance to the device, switching to CPAP, resolution of OSA after other adjunctive procedures, and significant weight loss [4]. While tracheostomy has been almost uniformly effective in relieving OSA, the chances of obstructive sleep apnea resolution allowing decannulation remain poor [4].

10.6 Complications

There have been multiple publications highlighting the inherent difficulties and complications associated with tracheostomies, but do not account specifically for OSA or the obese patient. These studies have reported a large range of potential complications from 4 to 40% [23]. Thatcher and Maisel [4] looked at 79 patients who underwent tracheostomy at a regional sleep disorder center and demonstrated that significant morbidity and mortality are low for the procedure. For the obese patient however, the rate of perioperative complications for open tracheostomy has been shown to be greater [18]. Body mass index was independently associated with increased risk of tracheostomy-related complications [24]. Multiple studies have shown not only a higher complication rate in the morbidly obese but also a higher mortality rate [23–25].

Complications can be categorized as intraoperative, early postoperative, and late postoperative. These complications can be further described as minor and major (or serious) events.

Bleeding can occur at any point of the procedure and within the early postoperative period. Minor bleeding is one of the most common early complications and can typically be controlled with local hemostasis maneuvers including the placement of Surgicel or topical thrombin. Major bleeding requires a return to the operating room and stabilization of the patient in order to prevent mortality from the procedure. An early sentinel bleed from a trachea-innominate artery fistula may provide an early warning of this devastating complication. Unfortunately, this is not always the case, and the patient may present with massive bleeding which is often associated with a high mortality rate.

The abnormal neck anatomy in the patient with OSA previously described in this chapter increases the risk of tube dislodgement or inadvertent decannulation. A cuff leak may occur due to cuff malfunctioning or due to loss of tracheal wall rigidity due to a poorly fitting tracheostomy tube. Selecting a proper tube size, as mentioned in this chapter, or exchange for a new tube will solve this issue. Tube obstruction can occur secondary to mucous plugging, blood clot within the tube, or obstruction from the tracheal wall. Infection at the stoma may occur and is managed with topical and systemic antibiotics. Drainage of multi-space infection resistant to medical management may require surgical intervention and additional IV antibiotics. Postoperative wound care is essential in order to prevent infection.

10.7 Summary

Tracheostomy continues to be a viable management option for patients with OSA who fail other interventions. One must take into consideration the anatomical differences in these patients including a posteriorly displaced airway due to increased adipose tissue and neck circumference. This patient population also has a higher likelihood of obesity, which adds to the complexity in performing tracheostomy. These challenges can be overcome with optimizing the surgical field with a proper setup, removing excess adipose tissue during the procedure, and proper tracheostomy tube selection. Postoperative education on tracheostomy care is also a must in order to facilitate a smooth discharge and ensure long-term patient compliance.

References

1. Kuhlo W, Doll E, Franck MC. [Successful management of Pickwickian syndrome using long-term tracheostomy]. Dtsch Med Wochenschr. 1969;94:1286.
2. Camacho M, Certal V, Brietzke SE, Holty J-EC, Guilleminault C, Capasso R. Tracheostomy as treatment for adult obstructive sleep apnea: a systematic review and meta-analysis. Laryngoscope. 2014;124:803.
3. Riley RW, Powell NB, Guilleminault C. Obstructive sleep apnea syndrome: a surgical protocol for dynamic upper airway reconstruction. J Oral Maxillofac Surg. 1993;51:742.
4. Thatcher GW, Maisel RH. The long-term evaluation of tracheostomy in the management of severe obstructive sleep apnea. Laryngoscope. 2003;113:201.
5. Fletcher EC, Schaaf JW, Miller J, Fletcher JG. Long-term cardiopulmonary sequelae in patients with sleep apnea and chronic lung disease. Am Rev Respir Dis. 1987;135:525.
6. Guilleminault C, Connolly SJ, Winkle RA. Cardiac arrhythmia and conduction disturbances during sleep in 400 patients with sleep apnea syndrome. Am J Cardiol. 1983;52:490.
7. He J, Kryger MH, Zorick FJ, Conway W, Roth T. Mortality and apnea index in obstructive sleep apnea. Experience in 385 male patients. Chest. 1988;94:9.
8. Calle EE, Thun MJ, Petrelli JM, Rodriguez C, Heath CWJ. Body-mass index and mortality in a prospective cohort of U.S. adults. N Engl J Med. 1999;341:1097.
9. Harris AT, Morell D, Bajaj Y, Martin-Hirsch DP. A discussion of airway and respiratory complications along with general considerations in obese patients. Int J Clin Pract. 2010;64:802.
10. Gross ND, Cohen JI, Andersen PE, Wax MK. "Defatting" tracheotomy in morbidly obese patients. Laryngoscope. 2002;112:1940.
11. Romero-Corral A, Caples SM, Lopez-Jimenez F, Somers VK. Interactions between obesity and obstructive sleep apnea: implications for treatment. Chest. 2010;137:711.
12. Young T, Palta M, Dempsey J, Skatrud J, Weber S, Badr S. The occurrence of sleep-disordered breathing among middle-aged adults. N Engl J Med. 1993;328:1230.
13. Bixler EO, Vgontzas AN, Ten Have T, Tyson K, Kales A. Effects of age on sleep apnea in men: I. prevalence and severity. Am J Respir Crit Care Med. 1998;157:144.
14. Bixler EO, Vgontzas AN, Lin HM, Ten Have T, Rein J, Vela-Bueno A, Kales A. Prevalence of sleep-disordered breathing in women: effects of gender. Am J Respir Crit Care Med. 2001;163:608.
15. Duran J, Esnaola S, Rubio R, Iztueta A. Obstructive sleep apnea-hypopnea and related clinical features in a population-based sample of subjects aged 30 to 70 yr. Am J Respir Crit Care Med. 2001;163:685.
16. Kim J, In K, Kim J, You S, Kang K, Shim J, Lee S, Lee J, Lee S, Park C, Shin C. Prevalence of sleep-disordered breathing in middle-aged Korean men and women. Am J Respir Crit Care Med. 2004;170:1108.
17. Sharma SK, Kumpawat S, Banga A, Goel A. Prevalence and risk factors of obstructive sleep apnea syndrome in a population of Delhi, India. Chest. 2006;130:149.
18. Cordes SR, Best AR, Hiatt KK. The impact of obesity on adult tracheostomy complication rate. Laryngoscope. 2015;125:105.
19. Kumar A, Camacho M, Capasso R. Quantitative assessment of an obstructive sleep apnea patient before and after tracheostomy: a case study. J Otol Rhinol. 2013;2:2.
20. Ankichetty S, Wong J, Chung F. A systematic review of the effects of sedatives and anesthetics in patients with obstructive sleep apnea. J Anaesthesiol Clin Pharmacol. 2011;27:447.
21. Lam KK, Kunder S, Wong J, Doufas AG, Chung F. Obstructive sleep apnea, pain, and opioids: is the riddle solved? Curr Opin Anaesthesiol. 2016;29:134.

22. Wolfe RM, Pomerantz J, Miller DE, Weiss-Coleman R, Solomonides T. Obstructive sleep apnea: preoperative screening and postoperative care. J Am Board Fam Med. 2016;29:263.
23. Fattahi T, Chafin C, Bunnell A. Tracheostomy in the morbidly obese: difficulties and challenges. J Oral Maxillofac Surg. 2017;75:1372.
24. El Solh AA, Jaafar W. A comparative study of the complications of surgical tracheostomy in morbidly obese critically ill patients. Crit Care. 2007;11:R3.
25. Darrat I, Yaremchuk K. Early mortality rate of morbidly obese patients after tracheotomy. Laryngoscope. 2008;118:2125.

Management of Pediatric Obstructive Sleep Apnea

11

Barry Steinberg, Rania A. Habib, and Yirae Ort

11.1 Introduction

Pediatric obstructive sleep apnea (OSA) remains controversial in the medical field. Not only does the definition of OSA change depending on the literature reviewed, but also the actual age group defined as the pediatric population varies. In 1996, the American Thoracic Society defined obstructive sleep apnea syndrome (OSAS) in children as a "disorder of breathing during sleep characterized by prolonged partial upper airway obstruction and/or intermittent complete obstruction (obstructive apnea) that disrupt normal ventilation during sleep and normal sleep patterns" [1]. The upper airway includes the nose, nasal passages, paranasal sinuses, pharynx, oral cavity, and the portion of the larynx above the vocal folds. OSA must be distinguished from primary snoring. Primary snoring is defined by the American Sleep Disorders Association as "snoring without obstructive sleep apnea, frequent arousal from sleep, or gas exchange abnormalities" [2, 3]. Gas exchange abnormalities refer to hypoxia, hypoxemia, hypercapnia, or hypopnea.

The general census among the specialists that treat pediatric OSA is that it is an underdiagnosed condition that causes significant morbidity and reduction in the quality of life when left untreated.

B. Steinberg (✉)
Department of Oral and Maxillofacial Surgery, College of Medicine, University of Florida—Jacksonville, Jacksonville, FL, USA

Wolfsons Children's Hospital, Jacksonville, FL, USA
e-mail: barry.steinberg@jax.ufl.edu

R. A. Habib
Department of Oral and Maxillofacial Surgery, School of Dentistry, Louisiana State University, New Orleans, LA, USA
e-mail: rhabib@lsuhsc.edu

Y. Ort
Facial Cosmetic Surgery, Bellevue, WA, USA

S. O. Salman (ed.), *Modern Management of Obstructive Sleep Apnea*,
https://doi.org/10.1007/978-3-030-11443-5_11

11.2 Epidemiology and Prevalence

The estimated overall prevalence of pediatric OSA is ~2–5% [4, 5]. Unfortunately, this percentage only includes patients who met the criteria for OSA based upon polysomnography. Snoring occurs in about 10% of pediatric patients [6]. Although snoring can be considered benign by itself, it can contribute to sleep-disordered breathing, especially when combined with obesity. Due to differences in practice, only about 10% of pediatric patients referred to the PCP for snoring are actually prescribed a sleep study. The prevalence of OSA is likely greatly underestimated because snoring is not present in all OSA patients, and such a small percentage of patients who snore actually receive a sleep study, the gold standard of the diagnosis of OSA [7, 8].

OSA is most common in preschool-aged children, aged 3–6. This is attributed to the size of the tonsils and adenoids relative to the posterior airway space and airway size [9]. The mean age of diagnosis is reported as 14 months ± 12 months. In this age group, OSA occurs equally in boys and girls and in highest prevalence among African Americans [4]. The frequency of OSA decreases after 9–10 years of age, with male predominance increasing after puberty [10].

The incidence of OSA increases in children diagnosed with craniofacial anomalies or syndromes. OSA in children with cleft lip and/or palate is 22–65%, 37–68% in syndromes with craniosynostosis, and 85% of children with Pierre Robin sequence [11–16].

11.3 Pathophysiology

The mechanisms by which the posterior airway obstruction occurs can be divided into two broad categories that include airway collapsibility and anatomic narrowing. Airway collapsibility can be caused by inflammation, hypotonia, tracheomalacia, and altered neuromotor reflexes. Pro-inflammatory cytokines that are increased in lymphoid tissue include TNF alpha, interleukin 6, and alpha 1. Inflammation may play a key role because it not only decreases the posterior airway space, but it also increases the risk of infection that causes collapse of the airway. Anatomic narrowing can occur anywhere in the respiratory tract and can be attributed to adeno-tonsillar hypertrophy, macroglossia, increased nasal resistance, craniofacial abnormalities, and lingual tonsil hypertrophy [17]. Lingual tonsil hypertrophy obliterates the vallecula and pushes the epiglottis posteriorly, which effectively narrows the airway. The craniofacial abnormalities that contribute to increasing the risk of OSA include retrognathia, micrognathia, midface hypoplasia, and abnormal anatomy of the cranial base. OSA is a complex condition, and it is important to remember that patients can possess multiple risk factors for developing OSA.

11.4 Risk Factors and Medical Conditions Associated with Pediatric OSA

11.4.1 Tonsillar and Adenoid Hypertrophy

The adenoids and tonsils reach peak growth relative to the size of the posterior nasopharynx and oropharynx during age 3–6 and can cause mechanical obstruction. Although adeno-tonsillar hypertrophy is thought to be the primary mechanism of upper airway obstruction in school-age children, studies have been unable to correlate the size of adeno-tonsillar hypertrophy to the degree of severity of OSA [18, 19].

11.4.2 Obesity

The prevalence of childhood obesity based on CDC data collected from 2011 to 2014 is 17%. The distribution includes 8.9% of 2–5-year-olds, 17.5% of 6–11-year-olds, and 20.5% of 12–19-year-olds [20]. The prevalence of OSA in obese pediatric patients approaches 50% [21]. This is attributed to increased neck circumference, intrathoracic pressure, leptin, and fatty submucosal infiltrates in the posterior airway space, as well as hypertrophy of the adenoids and lingual tonsils. Additionally, they also have decreased lung volumes and oxygen reserve [22]. In contrast to adults, however, the correlation between obesity and pediatric OSA is not very clear. Studies suggest there is an increased risk of OSA among obese adolescents aged 12 years and older; however, the risk of OSA was not significantly increased with increasing body mass among younger children [23].

11.4.3 Prematurity

Preterm babies are 3–5 times more likely to have OSA during childhood and two times as likely to develop OSA as an adult when compared to full-term babies. A recent retrospective study concluded that the negative impact of chronic lung disease of premature babies on gas exchange and lung volume combined with the abnormally decreased ventilatory drive all contribute to the development of OSA as they grow [24].

11.4.4 Craniofacial Deformities

Several congenital syndromes have various forms of disordered breathing or anatomic features that could contribute to OSA. These syndromes include but are not limited to Crouzon, Apert's syndrome, Pierre Robin sequence, Pfeiffer,

Treacher-Collins, Prader-Willi, Down syndrome (trisomy 21), Beckwith-Wiedemann syndrome, Klippel-Feil syndrome, Marfan's syndrome, and Fragile X [25, 26]. Among the craniofacial patients that undergo polysomnography, it was found that 22–65% of cleft lip ± palate, 40–60% of Apert/Crouzon/Pfeiffer craniosynostosis syndromes, and 85% of Pierre Robin sequence have OSA [11]. Craniofacial patients are complex because many have components of both central and obstructive sleep apnea [27]. Craniofacial dysmorphology in these patients often has key anatomic abnormalities that contribute to airway obstruction that include midface hypoplasia, choanal atresia, high and narrow palatal arch, macroglossia, glossoptosis, mandibular hypoplasia, microretrognathia, subglottic stenosis, laryngomalacia, tracheomalacia, and laryngeal atresia [28]. In addition, patients with craniofacial anomalies often have acute cranial base angles that correlate with increased risk of OSA [29].

OSA in children with craniofacial deformities is often multifactorial. A Down syndrome patient with trisomy 21 may have macroglossia, midface and mandibular hypoplasia, and hypotonia, which all contribute to posterior airway obstruction [30]. In Prader-Willi, the deleted chromosome 15 contributes to weak musculature due to hypotonia, poor feeding, and slow development. As these children age, they then develop constant hunger that leads to both obesity and insulin resistance. OSA in Prader-Willi patients could thus be attributed to hypotonia, obesity, and insulin resistance [31].

11.4.5 Neuromuscular Disorders

Children with neuromuscular disease suffer from pulmonary complications grouped into two main categories that include failure of the lung or failure of the respiratory pump [32]. Hypotonia of the muscles of the upper airway contributes to collapse of the posterior airway space during inspiration. Neuromuscular disease can produce narrowing of the posterior airway space on the level of the nasal and oropharyngeal area due to weakness of the pharyngeal and genioglossus muscles, respectively [33].

Other medical conditions associated with OSA in children include choanal stenosis, mucopolysaccharidosis, osteopetrosis, and sickle cell disease.

11.5 Clinical Presentation of Pediatric OSA

Nighttime symptoms include habitual snoring, witnessed apnea, frequent awakenings during sleep, night terrors, gasping for air, mouth breathing, neck hyperextension, secondary nocturnal enuresis, and frequent nocturnal awakenings. Daytime symptoms include lack of concentration, hyperactivity, inattention, restlessness, behavior problems, poor academic performance, daytime sleepiness, diaphoresis, nasal speech pattern, and mouth breathing. The consequences of obstructive sleep apnea in children manifest in various organ systems [34, 35].

11.5.1 Neurocognitive Sequelae

Several studies link pediatric OSA with a decrease in neurocognitive function that is often associated with decreased attention and/or concentration, hyperactivity, and aggressive behavior [36, 37]. The exact mechanisms by which OSA elicits neurocognitive deficits remain unclear. Research speculates that both sleep fragmentation and episodic hypoxia may lead to alterations within the neurochemical substrate of the prefrontal cortex with resultant executive dysfunction and neuronal cell loss [38, 39].

11.5.2 Cardiovascular Sequelae

Similar to adult patients, OSA can exert changes that affect the cardiovascular system in children. These adverse effects include systemic hypertension, changes in the left ventricular geometry, pulmonary hypertension, and endothelial dysfunction. Those changes are reflected in increased circulating levels of adhesion molecules and inflammatory responses within the microvasculature [40–43].

11.5.3 Weight Changes

While OSA in adults is strongly linked to obesity, weight changes in children with OSA can manifest either as obesity or as failure to thrive. Obesity can result from long-standing obstructive sleep apnea in association with insulin resistance and increased leptin levels resulting from lack of sleep. On the other hand, OSA can also cause increase work of breathing that causes the infant to burn calories in excess of those consumed and thus manifests as failure to thrive [44].

11.5.4 Insulin Resistance and Metabolic Syndrome

OSA, in the presence of obesity, increases the risk of developing metabolic syndrome in the pediatric population by increasing insulin resistance and lipid levels in the blood [45]. Leptin plays a role in regulating appetite, sleep, metabolic homeostasis, and respiratory control. Resistance to leptin is increased in pediatric patients, independent of the degree of obesity. Leptin acts as a respiratory stimulant in collaboration with central and peripheral chemoreceptors, so patients with leptin resistance have a weakened ventilatory response [46, 47].

11.5.5 Psychiatric Sequelae

Children with OSA experience decreased quality of life due to increased fatigue, irritability, impaired concentration, and depressed mood [48].

11.6 Diagnosis

Diagnosis of obstructive sleep apnea (OSA) in children versus adults is different in a few ways. A questionnaire-based screening in the pediatric population has low sensitivity and specificity—35% and 39%—respectively [49]. If a clinician has high suspicion that a child has OSA based on physical examination, further investigation and an appropriate referral to a specialist should be made. The presence of hyperplastic lymphoid tissues, large tongue, maxillary or mandibular hypoplasia, excessive overjet or crossbite, and obesity is suggestive of OSA in the presence of sleep disturbances and warrant further workup.

Overnight polysomnography is the gold standard for diagnosis; however, this procedure can often be difficult to perform in children due to poor cooperation with the attachment of monitoring devices and fear of sleeping in an unfamiliar environment. Polysomnography involves measuring several parameters including end-tidal CO_2, pulse oximetry, transcutaneous O_2 and CO_2 tensions (in infants and children <8 years), airflow at nose and mouth (pneumotachograph, thermistor), chest and abdominal wall motion (plethysmography), sleep state (EEG leads), electrooculogram, submental electromyogram (EMG study), electrocardiogram (ECG), and video monitoring with sound montage. Other alternative techniques such as nap polysomnography have been used in children, as it is shorter in duration and more convenient for the parent. However, this has a positive predictive value of 89% and a negative predictive value of 17%, which suggests that a child testing negative for OSA during a nap polysomnography should still undergo a more comprehensive evaluation and ideally an overnight polysomnography for definitive diagnosis if the patient's presentation strongly suggests OSA.

There are no standard imaging studies used in the diagnosis of OSA. Lateral cephalometric radiograph can demonstrate several indicators for higher likelihood of obstructive sleep apnea, such as posterior airway space, elongated soft palate, acute cranial base angles, and mandibular plane to hyoid distance. However, definitive correlation between these measurements alone and OSA has not been firmly established [50]. CT provides 3D images of the upper airway, allowing detailed views of the cross-sectional area, volume, and shape. Although some studies suggest CT scan for evaluating patients with OSA, it is not often used in pediatric population due to concerns with unnecessary radiation. It is worthy to note that lying in a supine position while awake does not duplicate the soft-tissue architecture produced in the altered neuromuscular activity found during sleep. Fiberoptic nasopharyngoscopy can be used as an adjunct to confirm the diagnosis and to identify the anatomic location and structural and/or functional abnormality that may contribute to obstructive sleep apnea. It requires patient cooperation; therefore, it serves greater diagnostic value in older children.

Polysomnographic criteria for defining OSA in children shares similarity to the criteria used with adults, but there are some significant differences. In adults, an apneic event is defined by the duration of the lack of breath which is 10 seconds. In children, an apnea event is classified by one or more missed breaths and is considered apnea even with the event lasts less than 10 seconds. Breath cycle, rather than time, is used in the children because the baseline pediatric respiratory rate is faster than that in adults until they reach late adolescence. Hypopnea is defined as ≥50% reduction in airflow measured by nasal air pressure transducer, accompanied by an arousal or ≥3% decrease in oxygen desaturation. This slightly varies from the criteria for adults, which is defined by ≥30% reduction in nasal airflow, accompanied by ≥4% oxygen desaturation [51].

Another factor that differs is the measurement of hypoventilation. For adults, sleep hypoventilation is defined as arterial $PCO_2 > 55$ mmHG for ≥ 10 minutes or an increase in arterial $PCO_2 \geq 10$ mmHg above the awake supine value. For pediatric patients, hypoventilation is defined as arterial $PCO_2 > 50$ mmHg for >25% of total sleep time or an arterial $PCO_2 > 53$ mmHg during any period of total sleep time [52].

The criteria for defining OSA in the pediatric population has a much lower threshold than adults. An apnea-hypopnea index (AHI) >1.5 is considered abnormal in children where in adults an abnormal AHI is >5. Although there are several different indices as well as varying opinions among the experts, most sleep centers define the severity of OSA in children using the following parameters: AHI < 1 normal, AHI 1.5 ≤ 5 mild OSA, AHI 5 ≤ 10 moderate OSA, AHI > 10 severe OSA [53].

11.7 Management

The most common first-line treatment for children with OSA is adenotonsillectomy. Meta-analysis literature shows the success rate of tonsillectomy and adenoidectomy to be approximately 79–85% in the pediatric population [54, 55]. However, long-term outcome studies in patients after adenotonsillectomy are lacking, and it is often difficult to identify whether recurrence or persistence of OSA occurs due to other factors such as obesity or existing lingual tonsil hypertrophy [56].

A less commonly used surgical treatment for pediatric OSA is uvulopalatopharyngoplasty (UPPP). This is because children, with or without sleep apnea, do not demonstrate as much redundant palatopharyngeal tissue as adults. However, UPPP is found to have some benefit in children with abnormal upper airway neuromuscular tone. This is seen in children with cerebral palsy, Down syndrome, or high Mallampati score due to redundant lateral pharyngeal tissue [57].

A reasonable option in non-surgical candidates is continuous positive airway pressure (CPAP). Depending on the facial structure and size of the child, CPAP can be administered via facial mask as in adults or via nasal masks. Due to logistical issues, nasal CPAP is generally the preferred method in most pediatric patients [58]. Successful treatment requires parental support in addition to patient compliance and frequent clinician assessment. Children with poor parental support and those with behavior problems that cannot tolerate the CPAP may thus not benefit from CPAP as a treatment modality.

Children with mild OSA may benefit from a reduction of upper airway inflammation using topical intranasal application of corticosteroids [59]. Similarly, montelukast receptor blocker was found to be effective in reducing symptoms in children with mild OSA [60]. Since appropriate duration of these treatments and their

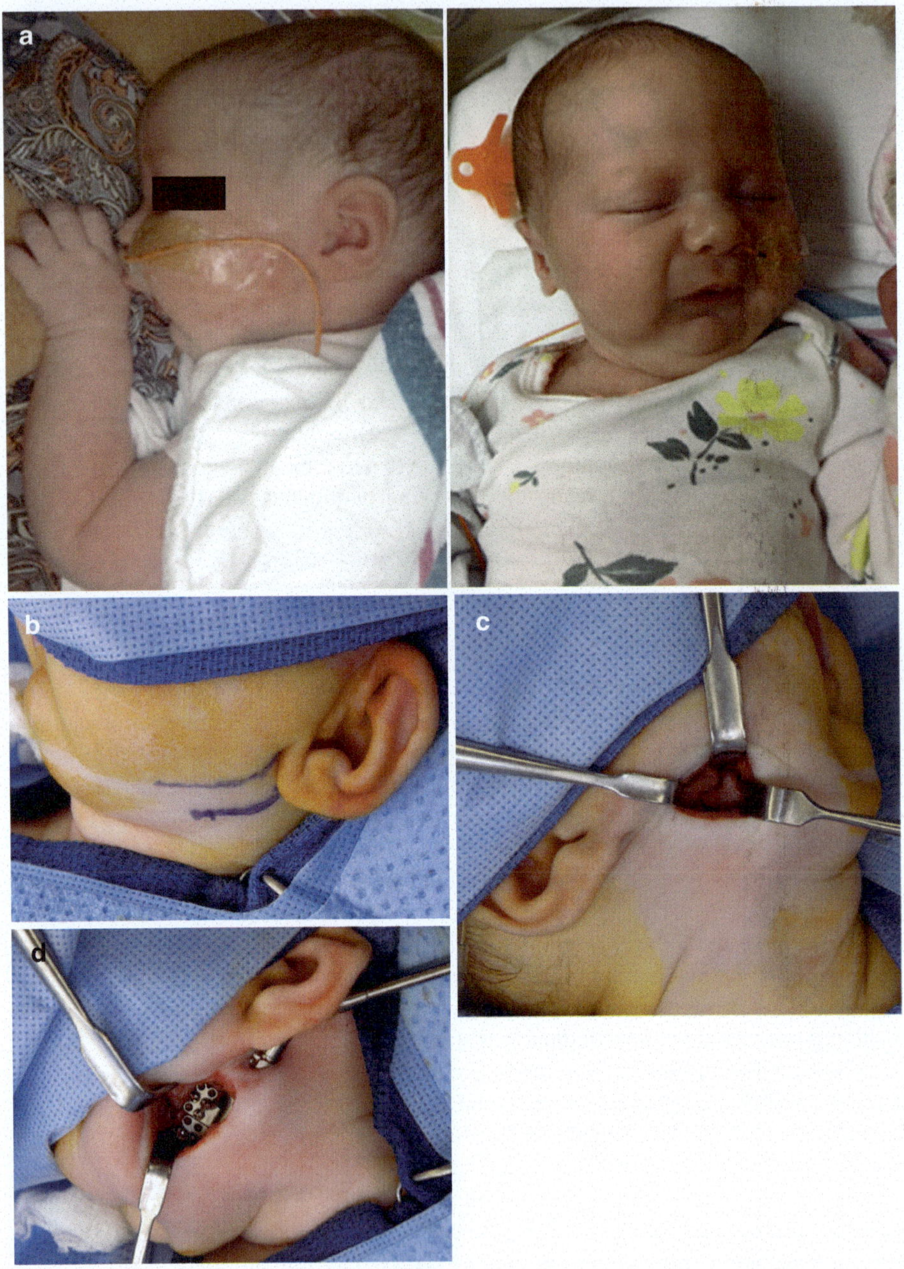

Fig. 11.1 (**a**) Preoperative photos of an infant with OSA and feeding problems due to microretrognathia and Pierre Robin Sequence. Note that the mandible is hypoplastic and retrognathic. (**b**) Intraoperative marking outlining the inferior border of the mandible and incision site. (**c**) Mandibular osteotomy. (**d**) Mandibular distractor placement. (**e**) Post-operative photographs demonstrating advancement of the mandible into a prognathic position. (**f**) Intraoperative photograph demonstrating good bony consolidation following removal of mandibular distractor

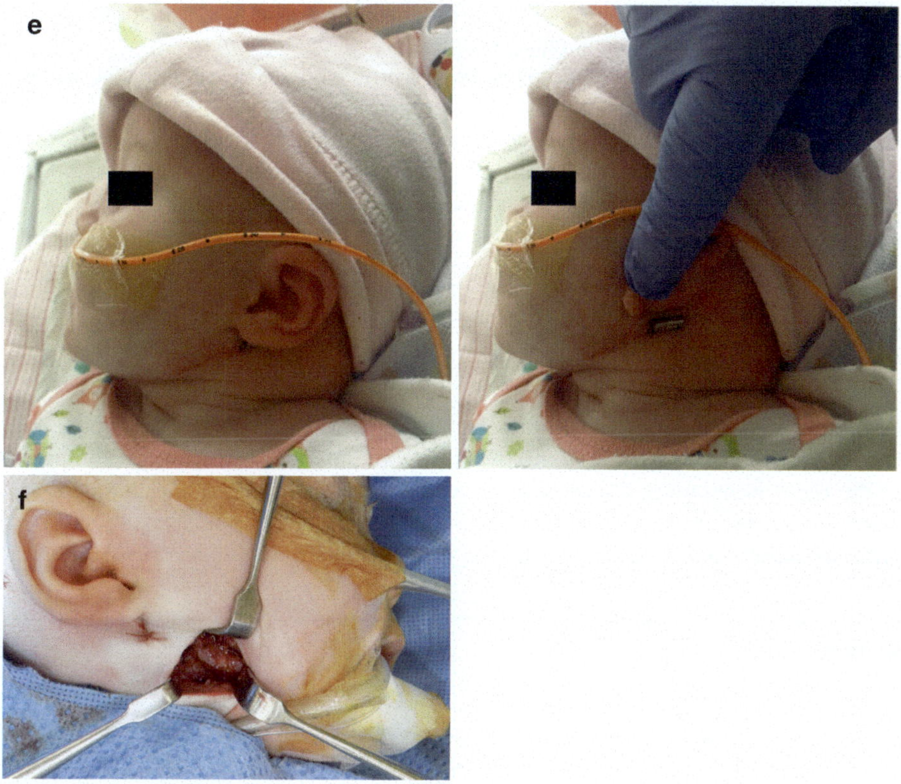

Fig. 11.1 (continued)

long-term effects have not been established, these are considered adjuncts to therapy and are not recommended as first line treatment for OSA.

Severe OSA due to certain craniomaxillofacial skeletal abnormalities may benefit from distraction osteogenesis (DO). The goal of DO is to diminish the need for tracheostomy or to help in early decannulation in patients who already have a surgical airway. Meta-analysis studies in the literature suggest the success rate of mandibular DO for treatment of pediatric OSA is approximately 90–96% [61]. Indications for mandibular DO in the pediatric population include severe hypoplasia, failure of nonsurgical airway such as CPAP, or failure of previous surgical intervention. Distraction osteogenesis is rarely the first-line treatment modality. Many patients with non-syndromic micrognathia will undergo catch-up growth, outgrowing their airway issues and obviating the need for surgery [62]. Complications of mandibular DO include vector control, which may lead to poor occlusal or functional relationship potentiating the need for secondary jaw surgery later in life. Other complications include TMJ trauma or ankylosis, facial asymmetry, inadequate consolidation, and relapse [63]. Figure 11.1a–f depicts the treatment sequence for an infant diagnosed with Pierre Robin sequence who had feeding difficulty and

OSA secondary to microretrognathia. After successful mandibular distraction, the patient resumed oral feeds and had resolution of OSA symptoms.

The most definitive treatment to establish a protected airway remains the tracheostomy. It is associated with numerous complications that include but are not limited to scars, granulation tissue, accidental decannulation, tracheal stenosis, tube occlusion and fistula. In a retrospective study reviewing the complications in pediatric tracheostomies, Carr et al. found that 77% had complications of which 43% were considered serious [64]. Trachestomy should thus be reserved for the most severe cases of OSA that cannot be successfully treated with any other methods.

11.8 Summary

Pediatric OSA has many similarities to that described in the adult population. However, it tends to be more complex with more potential causes when compared to the older population. Differences in anatomy and neurologic development are factors add to these age related variations. The treatment paradigm also is somewhat different with remaining growth entering into the equation.

References

1. Standards and indications for cardiopulmonary sleep studies in children. Am J Respir Crit Care Med. 1996;153:866–78. https://doi.org/10.1164/ajrccm.153.2.8564147.
2. A.S.D. Association. International classification of sleep disorders, revised: diagnostic and coding manual. Rochester, MN: American Sleep Disorders Association; 1997.
3. Farber JM. Clinical practice guideline: diagnosis and management of childhood obstructive sleep apnea syndrome. Pediatrics. 2002;110:1255–7.
4. Redline S, Tishler PV, Schluchter M, Aylor J, Clark K, Graham G. Risk factors for sleep-disordered breathing in children. Associations with obesity, race, and respiratory problems. Am J Respir Crit Care Med. 1999;159:1527–32. https://doi.org/10.1164/ajrccm.159.5.9809079.
5. Marcus CL, Brooks LJ, Draper KA, Gozal D, Halbower AC, Jones J, Schechter MS, Ward SD, Sheldon SH, Shiffman RN, Lehmann C, Spruyt K, American Academy of Pediatrics. Diagnosis and management of childhood obstructive sleep apnea syndrome. Pediatrics. 2012;130:e714–55. https://doi.org/10.1542/peds.2012-1672.
6. Hultcrantz E, Lofstrand-Tidestrom B, Ahlquist-Rastad J. The epidemiology of sleep related breathing disorder in children. Int J Pediatr Otorhinolaryngol. 1995;32 Suppl:S63–6. https://doi.org/10.1016/0165-5876(94)01144-M.
7. Lumeng JC, Chervin RD. Epidemiology of pediatric obstructive sleep apnea. Proc Am Thorac Soc. 2008;5:242–52. https://doi.org/10.1513/pats.200708-135MG.
8. Mitchell RB, Pereira KD, Friedman NR. Sleep-disordered breathing in children: survey of current practice. Laryngoscope. 2006;116(6):956–8. https://doi.org/10.1097/01.MLG.0000216413.22408.FD.
9. Jeans WD, Fernando DC, Maw AR, Leighton BC. A longitudinal study of the growth of the nasopharynx and its contents in normal children. Br J Radiol. 1981;54:117–21. https://doi.org/10.1259/0007-1285-54-638-117.
10. Goodwin JL, Babar SI, Kaemingk KL, Rosen GM, Morgan WJ, Sherrill DL, Quan SF, Tucson Children's Assessment of Sleep Apnea Study. Symptoms related to sleep-disordered breathing in white and hispanic children: the Tucson Children's Assessment of Sleep Apnea study. Chest. 2003;124:196–203. https://doi.org/10.1378/chest.124.1.196.

11. Garg RK, Afifi AM, Garland CB, Sanchez R, Mount DL. Pediatric obstructive sleep apnea: consensus, controversy, and craniofacial considerations. Plast Reconstr Surg. 2017;140:987–97. https://doi.org/10.1097/PRS.0000000000003752.
12. MacLean JE, Fitzsimons D, Fitzgerald DA, Waters KA. The spectrum of sleep-disordered breathing symptoms and respiratory events in infants with cleft lip and/or palate. Arch Dis Child. 2012;97:1058–63. https://doi.org/10.1136/archdischild-2012-302104.
13. Driessen C, Mathijssen IM, De Groot MR, Joosten KF. Does central sleep apnea occur in children with syndromic craniosynostosis? Respir Physiol Neurobiol. 2012;181:321–5. https://doi.org/10.1016/j.resp.2012.03.017.
14. Bannink N, Maliepaard M, Raat H, Joosten KF, Mathijssen IM. Obstructive sleep apnea-specific quality of life and behavioral problems in children with syndromic craniosynostosis. J Dev Behav Pediatr. 2011;32:233–8. https://doi.org/10.1097/DBP.0b013e318206d5e3.
15. Anderson IC, Sedaghat AR, McGinley BM, Redett RJ, Boss EF, Ishman SL. Prevalence and severity of obstructive sleep apnea and snoring in infants with Pierre Robin sequence. Cleft Palate Craniofac J. 2011;48:614–8. https://doi.org/10.1597/10-100.
16. MacLean JE, Hayward P, Fitzgerald DA, Waters K. Cleft lip and/or palate and breathing during sleep. Sleep Med Rev. 2009;13:345–54. https://doi.org/10.1016/j.smrv.2009.03.001.
17. DelRosso LM. Epidemiology and diagnosis of pediatric obstructive sleep apnea. Curr Probl Pediatr Adolesc Health Care. 2016;46:2–6. https://doi.org/10.1016/j.cppeds.2015.10.009.
18. Tang A, Benke JR, Cohen AP, Ishman SL. Influence of tonsillar size on OSA improvement in children undergoing adenotonsillectomy. Otolaryngol Head Neck Surg. 2015;153:281–5. https://doi.org/10.1177/0194599815583459.
19. Shen L, Zheng B, Lin Z, Xu Y, Yang Z. Tailoring therapy to improve the treatment of children with obstructive sleep apnea according to grade of adenotonsillar hypertrophy. Int J Pediatr Otorhinolaryngol. 2015;79:493–8. https://doi.org/10.1016/j.ijporl.2015.01.005.
20. Center for Disease Control, Childhood Obesity Data. (n.d.). https://www.cdc.gove/obesity/data/childhood.html.
21. Verhulst SL, Van Gaal L, De Backer W, Desager K. The prevalence, anatomical correlates and treatment of sleep-disordered breathing in obese children and adolescents. Sleep Med Rev. 2008;12:339–46. https://doi.org/10.1016/j.smrv.2007.11.002.
22. Blechner M, Williamson AA. Consequences of obstructive sleep apnea in children. Curr Probl Pediatr Adolesc Health Care. 2016;46:19–26. https://doi.org/10.1016/j.cppeds.2015.10.007.
23. Kohler MJ, Thormaehlen S, Kennedy JD, Pamula Y, van den Heuvel CJ, Lushington K, Martin AJ. Differences in the association between obesity and obstructive sleep apnea among children and adolescents. J Clin Sleep Med. 2009;5:506–11.
24. Armoni Domany K, Hossain MM, Nava-Guerra L, Khoo MC, McConnell K, Carroll JL, Xu Y, DiFrancesco M, Amin RS. Cardioventilatory control in preterm born children and the risk of obstructive sleep apnea. Am J Respir Crit Care Med. 2018;197(12):1596–603. https://doi.org/10.1164/rccm.201708-1700OC.
25. Boston M, Rutter MJ. Current airway management in craniofacial anomalies. Curr Opin Otolaryngol Head Neck Surg. 2003;11:428–32.
26. Palaiologos G, Felig P. Effects of ketone bodies on amino acid metabolism in isolated rat diaphragm. Biochem J. 1976;154:709–16.
27. Mass E, Brin I, Belostoky L, Maayan C, Gadoth N. A cephalometric evaluation of craniofacial morphology in familial dysautonomia. Cleft Palate Craniofac J. 1998;35:120–6. https://doi.org/10.1597/1545-1569_1998_035_0120_ACEOCM_2.3.CO_2.
28. Cielo CM, Marcus CL. Obstructive sleep apnoea in children with craniofacial syndromes. Paediatr Respir Rev. 2015;16:189–96. https://doi.org/10.1016/j.prrv.2014.11.003.
29. Steinberg B, Fraser B. The cranial base in obstructive sleep apnea. J Oral Maxillofac Surg. 1995;53:1150–4. https://doi.org/10.1016/0278-2391(95)90621-5.
30. Rosen D. Management of obstructive sleep apnea associated with down syndrome and other craniofacial dysmorphologies. Curr Opin Pulm Med. 2011;17:431–6. https://doi.org/10.1097/MCP.0b013e32834ba9c0.

31. Sedky K, Bennett DS, Pumariega A. Prader Willi syndrome and obstructive sleep apnea: co-occurrence in the pediatric population. J Clin Sleep Med. 2014;10:403–9. https://doi.org/10.5664/jcsm.3616.
32. Allen J. Pulmonary complications of neuromuscular disease: a respiratory mechanics perspective. Paediatr Respir Rev. 2010;11:18–23. https://doi.org/10.1016/j.prrv.2009.10.002.
33. Eikermann M, Vogt FM, Herbstreit F, Vahid-Dastgerdi M, Zenge MO, Ochterbeck C, de Greiff A, Peters J. The predisposition to inspiratory upper airway collapse during partial neuromuscular blockade. Am J Respir Crit Care Med. 2007;175:9–15. https://doi.org/10.1164/rccm.200512-1862OC.
34. Gozal D. Obstructive sleep apnea in children: implications for the developing central nervous system. Semin Pediatr Neurol. 2008;15:100–6. https://doi.org/10.1016/j.spen.2008.03.006.
35. Tan H-L, Gozal D, Kheirandish-Gozal L. Obstructive sleep apnea in children: a critical update. Nat Sci Sleep. 2013;5:109–23. https://doi.org/10.2147/NSS.S51907.
36. Bourke R, Anderson V, Yang JS, Jackman AR, Killedar A, Nixon GM, Davey MJ, Walker AM, Trinder J, Horne RS. Cognitive and academic functions are impaired in children with all severities of sleep-disordered breathing. Sleep Med. 2011;12:489–96. https://doi.org/10.1016/j.sleep.2010.11.010.
37. Miano S, Paolino MC, Urbano A, Parisi P, Massolo AC, Castaldo R, Villa MP. Neurocognitive assessment and sleep analysis in children with sleep-disordered breathing. Clin Neurophysiol. 2011;122:311–9. https://doi.org/10.1016/j.clinph.2010.06.019.
38. Halbower AC, Degaonkar M, Barker PB, Earley CJ, Marcus CL, Smith PL, Prahme MC, Mahone EM. Childhood obstructive sleep apnea associates with neuropsychological deficits and neuronal brain injury. PLoS Med. 2006;3:e301. https://doi.org/10.1371/journal.pmed.0030301.
39. Beebe DW, Gozal D. Obstructive sleep apnea and the prefrontal cortex: towards a comprehensive model linking nocturnal upper airway obstruction to daytime cognitive and behavioral deficits. J Sleep Res. 2002;11:1–16. https://doi.org/10.1046/j.1365-2869.2002.00289.x.
40. O'Brien LM, Serpero LD, Tauman R, Gozal D. Plasma adhesion molecules in children with sleep-disordered breathing. Chest. 2006;129:947–53. https://doi.org/10.1378/chest.129.4.947.
41. Amin RS, Kimball TR, Kalra M, Jeffries JL, Carroll JL, Bean JA, Witt SA, Glascock BJ, Daniels SR. Left ventricular function in children with sleep-disordered breathing. Am J Cardiol. 2005;95:801–4. https://doi.org/10.1016/j.amjcard.2004.11.044.
42. Marcus CL, Greene MG, Carroll JL. Blood pressure in children with obstructive sleep apnea. Am J Respir Crit Care Med. 1998;157:1098–103. https://doi.org/10.1164/ajrccm.157.4.9704080.
43. Alexander RW. Inflammation and coronary artery disease. N Engl J Med. 1994;331:468–9. https://doi.org/10.1056/NEJM199408183310709.
44. Freezer NJ, Bucens IK, Robertson CF. Obstructive sleep apnoea presenting as failure to thrive in infancy. J Paediatr Child Health. 1995;31:172–5.
45. Waters KA, Sitha S, O'brien LM, Bibby S, de Torres C, Vella S, de la Eva R. Follow-up on metabolic markers in children treated for obstructive sleep apnea. Am J Respir Crit Care Med. 2006;174:455–60. https://doi.org/10.1164/rccm.200401-110OC.
46. Myers MG, Cowley MA, Munzberg H. Mechanisms of leptin action and leptin resistance. Annu Rev Physiol. 2008;70:537–56. https://doi.org/10.1146/annurev.physiol.70.113006.100707.
47. Polotsky VY, Smaldone MC, Scharf MT, Li J, Tankersley CG, Smith PL, Schwartz AR, O'Donnell CP. Impact of interrupted leptin pathways on ventilatory control. J Appl Physiol (Bethesda, Md 1985). 2004;96:991–8. https://doi.org/10.1152/japplphysiol.00926.2003.
48. Hayflick L. Current theories of biological aging. Fed Proc. 1975;34:9–13. http://www.ncbi.nlm.nih.gov/pubmed/1088947.
49. Brouilette R, Hanson D, David R, Klemka L, Szatkowski A, Fernbach S, Hunt C. A diagnostic approach to suspected obstructive sleep apnea in children. J Pediatr. 1984;105:10–4.
50. Miles PG, Vig PS, Weyant RJ, Forrest TD, Rockette HE Jr. Craniofacial structure and obstructive sleep apnea syndrome—a qualitative analysis and meta-analysis of the literature. Am J Orthod Dentofac Orthop. 1996;109:163–72. https://doi.org/10.1016/S0889-5406(96)70177-4.

51. Accardo JA, Shults J, Leonard MB, Traylor J, Marcus CL. Differences in overnight polysomnography scores using the adult and pediatric criteria for respiratory events in adolescents. Sleep. 2010;33:1333–9. https://doi.org/10.1093/sleep/33.10.1333.
52. Berry RB, Budhiraja R, Gottlieb DJ, Gozal D, Iber C, Kapur VK, Marcus CL, Mehra R, Parthasarathy S, Quan SF, Redline S, Strohl KP, Davidson Ward SL, Tangredi MM, A.A. of S. Medicine. Rules for scoring respiratory events in sleep: update of the 2007 AASM manual for the scoring of sleep and associated events. Deliberations of the sleep apnea definitions task force of the American Academy of sleep medicine. J Clin Sleep Med. 2012;8:597–619. https://doi.org/10.5664/jcsm.2172.
53. Mitchell RB. Adenotonsillectomy for obstructive sleep apnea in children: outcome evaluated by pre- and postoperative polysomnography. Laryngoscope. 2007;117:1844–54. https://doi.org/10.1097/MLG.0b013e318123ee56.
54. Mitchell RB, Kelly J. Outcome of adenotonsillectomy for severe obstructive sleep apnea in children. Int J Pediatr Otorhinolaryngol. 2004;68:1375–9. https://doi.org/10.1016/j.ijporl.2004.04.026.
55. Lipton AJ, Gozal D. Treatment of obstructive sleep apnea in children: do we really know how? Sleep Med Rev. 2003;7:61–80. https://doi.org/10.1053/smrv.2001.0256.
56. Lin AC, Koltai PJ. Persistent pediatric obstructive sleep apnea and lingual tonsillectomy. Otolaryngol Head Neck Surg. 2009;141:81–5. https://doi.org/10.1016/j.otohns.2009.03.011.
57. Anand H, Roberts PJ, Badman G, Dixon AJ, Collins JF. Novel kainic acid analogues. Effects on cyclic GMP content of adult rat cerebellar slices. Biochem Pharmacol. 1986;35:409–15. https://doi.org/10.1016/0006-2952(86)90213-3.
58. O'Donnell AR, Bjornson CL, Bohn SG, Kirk VG. Compliance rates in children using noninvasive continuous positive airway pressure. Sleep. 2006;29:651–8.
59. Goldbart AD, Veling MC, Goldman JL, Li RC, Brittian KR, Gozal D. Glucocorticoid receptor subunit expression in adenotonsillar tissue of children with obstructive sleep apnea. Pediatr Res. 2005;57:232–6. https://doi.org/10.1203/01.PDR.0000150722.34561.E6.
60. Brouillette RT, Manoukian JJ, Ducharme FM, Oudjhane K, Earle LG, Ladan S, Morielli A. Efficacy of fluticasone nasal spray for pediatric obstructive sleep apnea. J Pediatr. 2001;138:838–44. https://doi.org/10.1067/mpd.2001.114474.
61. Tahiri Y, Viezel-Mathieu A, Aldekhayel S, Lee J, Gilardino M. The effectiveness of mandibular distraction in improving airway obstruction in the pediatric population. Plast Reconstr Surg. 2014;133:352e–9e. https://doi.org/10.1097/01.prs.0000438049.29258.a8.
62. Figueroa AA, Glupker TJ, Fitz MG, BeGole EA. Mandible, tongue, and airway in Pierre Robin sequence: a longitudinal cephalometric study. Cleft Palate Craniofac J. 1991;28:425–34. https://doi.org/10.1597/1545-1569(1991)028_0425:MTAAIP_2.3.CO_2.
63. Bouchard C, Troulis MJ, Kaban LB. Management of obstructive sleep apnea: role of distraction osteogenesis. Oral Maxillofac Surg Clin North Am. 2009;21:459–75. https://doi.org/10.1016/j.coms.2009.07.001.
64. Carr MM, Poje CP, Kingston L, Keilma D, Heard C. Complications in pediatric tracheostomies. Laryngoscope. 2001;111:1925–8.

The manufacturer's authorised representative in the EU is Springer Nature Customer Service Centre GmbH, Europaplatz 3, 69115 Heidelberg, Germany. If you have any concerns regarding our products, please contact ProductSafety@springernature.com

Printed and bound by CPI Group (UK) Ltd, Croydon, CR0 4YY
05/10/2026
02228160-0001